VOLUME ONE HUNDRED AND SIXTEEN

ADVANCES IN PARASITOLOGY

Accomplishment of Malaria Elimination in the People's Republic of China

VOLUME ONE HUNDRED AND SIXTEEN

ADVANCES IN PARASITOLOGY

Accomplishment of Malaria Elimination in the People's Republic of China

Edited by

MARCEL TANNER
Swiss Tropical and Public Health Institute;
University of Basel, Basel, Switzerland

JIAN-HAI YIN
National Institute of Parasitic Diseases, Chinese Center for Disease Control and Prevention (Chinese Center for Tropical Diseases Research),
NHC Key Laboratory of Parasite and Vector Biology,
WHO Collaborating Center for Tropical Diseases, National Center for International Research on Tropical Diseases

XIAO-NONG ZHOU
National Institute of Parasitic Diseases, Chinese Center for Disease Control and Prevention (Chinese Center for Tropical Diseases Research),
NHC Key Laboratory of Parasite and Vector Biology,
WHO Collaborating Center for Tropical Diseases, National Center for International Research on Tropical Diseases;
School of Global Health, Chinese Center for Tropical Diseases Research, Shanghai Jiao Tong University School of Medicine, Shanghai, PR China

ELSEVIER

ACADEMIC PRESS
An imprint of Elsevier

Academic Press is an imprint of Elsevier
125 London Wall, London EC2Y 5AS, United Kingdom
The Boulevard, Langford Lane, Kidlington, Oxford OX5 1GB, United Kingdom
50 Hampshire Street, 5th Floor, Cambridge, MA 02139, United States
525 B Street, Suite 1650, San Diego, CA 92101, United States

First edition 2022

ISBN: 978-0-323-95256-9
ISSN: 0065-308X

For information on all Academic Press publications
visit our website at https://www.elsevier.com/books-and-journals

Publisher: Zoe Kruze
Acquisitions Editor: Ashlie M. Jackman
Developmental Editor: Cindy Angelita Gardose
Production Project Manager: Abdulla Sait
Cover Designer: Christian Bilbow

Typeset by STRAIVE, India

Contents

Contributors ix
A malaria-free China: global importance and key experience xv

1. Case-based malaria surveillance and response: implementation of 1-3-7 approach in Jiangsu Province, China **1**
Yuanyuan Cao, Guangyu Lu, Huayun Zhou, Weiming Wang, Yaobao Liu, Mengmeng Yang, Cheng Liang, Guoding Zhu, and Jun Cao

1. Introduction 2
2. Background 3
3. Needs of intensive malaria surveillance and response approach 10
4. Implementation of malaria 1-3-7 surveillance and response approach in Jiangsu Province 15
5. Challenges for implementing malaria 1-3-7 approach in Jiangsu Province 20
6. Lessons learned from implementing malaria 1-3-7 approach in Jiangsu Province 23
7. Conclusions 28

Acknowledgements 28
References 28

2. Historical review of malaria control and elimination in the border areas of China: A case study of Yunnan Province **33**
Hui Liu, Yao-Wu Zhou, Yan Deng, Zu-Rui Lin, Cang-Lin Zhang, Qi-Yan Chen, Chun Wei, Kai-Xia Duan, Hong-Ning Zhou, and Jian-wei Xu

1. Introduction 34
2. Background 35
3. Malaria control from hyperendemicity to elimination 36
4. Experiences 51
5. Lessons 58
6. Challenges and recommendations 61
7. Conclusions 64

Acknowledgements 65
References 65

3. Surveillance and response systems driving malaria elimination in the mountain areas of Hainan Province **69**

Yuchun Li, Shanqing Wang, Ximin Hu, Yingjuan Huang, Renqiang Chen, Minchan Lin, Huanzhi Xu, Rongshen Ye, Datian Zhan, Shaoling Huang, Ji Zhen, Xiaodan Wen, Guoyi Wang, Yong Liu, Haishan Li, Zaichun Zheng, Jian Wang, Wen Zeng, Feng Meng, Xiaoming Huang, Guangze Wang, Bing Yang, and Yan Chen

1. Introduction 70
2. Background 72
3. The malaria surveillance and response system for forest goers in Hainan 88
4. Ongoing challenges and responses in forest goers after malaria elimination in Hainan Province 108

Acknowledgements 109
References 110

4. Mass drug administration in response to vivax malaria resurgence in Anhui Province of Huanghuai Plain, China **115**

Xian Xu, Jian-Jun Wang, Jing-Jing Jiang, Tao Zhang, Xiao-Feng Lv, Shu-Qi Wang, Zi-Jian Liu, Wei-Dong Li, and Xue-Chun Lu

1. Introduction 116
2. Background 117
3. Designing the focal MDA 121
4. Implementation of focal MDA 133
5. Other malaria control measures 141
6. Effectiveness of the response to the resurgence 144
7. Conclusions and perspectives 147

Acknowledgements 149
References 150

5. One Health approach to improve the malaria elimination programme in Henan Province **153**

Ying Liu, Zhi-Quan He, Dan Wang, Ya-Bo Hu, Dan Qian, Cheng-Yun Yang, Rui-min Zhou, Su-Hua Li, De-Ling Lu, and Hong-Wei Zhang

1. Introduction 155
2. One Health approach applied in malaria control programme 159
3. The elimination of malaria with One Health approach in Henan Province 160
4. Case studies on implementation of One Health approach in malaria control in Henan Province 166

5. Introduction of malaria control technologies supported by One Health approach 170
6. One Health approach applied in prevention of malaria retransmission 171
7. Lessons learnt from malaria control and elimination in Henan Province 179
8. Conclusions and perspectives 182
Acknowledgements 183
References 183

6. Research and development of traditional medicines in low- and middle-income countries: A case study of artemisinin discovery in China 187

Guang-qi Liu, Yan Xie, Yi-nuo Sun, Kai-xuan Zhang, Ji-yan Maa, and Yang-mu Huang

1. Introduction 188
2. Global and Chinese background 189
3. Research and development history of artemisinin 191
4. Conclusions and perspectives 205
Acknowledgements 207
References 207

Contributors

Jun Cao
Key Laboratory of National Health Commission (NHC) on Parasitic Disease Control and Prevention, Jiangsu Provincial Key Laboratory on Parasite and Vector Control Technology, Jiangsu Institute of Parasitic Diseases, Wuxi; Center for Global Health, School of Public Health, Nanjing Medical University, Nanjing, Jiangsu, PR China

Yuanyuan Cao
Key Laboratory of National Health Commission (NHC) on Parasitic Disease Control and Prevention, Jiangsu Provincial Key Laboratory on Parasite and Vector Control Technology, Jiangsu Institute of Parasitic Diseases, Wuxi, Jiangsu, PR China

Qi-Yan Chen
Yunnan Institute of Parasitic Diseases, Yunnan Provincial Centre of Malaria Research, Yunnan Provincial Key Laboratory of Vector-borne Diseases Control and Research, Yunnan Institute of Parasitic Diseases Innovative Team of Key Techniques for Vector Borne Disease Control and Prevention, Training Base of International Scientific Exchange and Education in Tropical Diseases for South and Southeast Asia, Puer, Yunnan, PR China

Renqiang Chen
Sanya City Center for Disease Control & Prevention, Sanya, Hainan, PR China

Yan Chen
Hainan Provincial Center for Disease Control & Prevention, Haikou, Hainan, PR China

Yan Deng
Yunnan Institute of Parasitic Diseases, Yunnan Provincial Centre of Malaria Research, Yunnan Provincial Key Laboratory of Vector-borne Diseases Control and Research, Yunnan Institute of Parasitic Diseases Innovative Team of Key Techniques for Vector Borne Disease Control and Prevention, Training Base of International Scientific Exchange and Education in Tropical Diseases for South and Southeast Asia, Puer, Yunnan, PR China

Kai-Xia Duan
Yunnan Institute of Parasitic Diseases, Yunnan Provincial Centre of Malaria Research, Yunnan Provincial Key Laboratory of Vector-borne Diseases Control and Research, Yunnan Institute of Parasitic Diseases Innovative Team of Key Techniques for Vector Borne Disease Control and Prevention, Training Base of International Scientific Exchange and Education in Tropical Diseases for South and Southeast Asia, Puer, Yunnan, PR China

Zhi-Quan He
Henan Center for Disease Control and Prevention, Zhengzhou, Henan, PR China

Ximin Hu
Hainan Provincial Center for Disease Control & Prevention, Haikou, Hainan, PR China

Ya-Bo Hu
Zhengzhou University, Zhengzhou, Henan, PR China

Shaoling Huang
Wanning City Center for Disease Control & Prevention, Wanning, Hainan, PR China

Xiaoming Huang
Hainan Provincial Center for Disease Control & Prevention, Haikou, Hainan, PR China

Yang-mu Huang
Department of Global Health, Peking University School of Public Health; Institute for Global Health, Peking University, Beijing, PR China

Yingjuan Huang
Sanya City Center for Disease Control & Prevention, Sanya, Hainan, PR China

Jing-Jing Jiang
Anhui Provincial Center for Disease Control and Prevention, Anhui, PR China

Christian Lengeler
Swiss Tropical and Public Health Institute; University of Basel, Basel, Switzerland

Haishan Li
Ledong County Center for Disease Control & Prevention, Ledong, Hainan, PR China

Su-Hua Li
Henan Center for Disease Control and Prevention, Zhengzhou, Henan, PR China

Wei-Dong Li
Anhui Provincial Center for Disease Control and Prevention, Anhui, PR China

Yuchun Li
Hainan Provincial Center for Disease Control & Prevention, Haikou, Hainan, PR China

Cheng Liang
Key Laboratory of National Health Commission (NHC) on Parasitic Disease Control and Prevention, Jiangsu Provincial Key Laboratory on Parasite and Vector Control Technology, Jiangsu Institute of Parasitic Diseases, Wuxi, Jiangsu, PR China

Minchan Lin
Wuzhishan City Center for Disease Control & Prevention, Wuzhishan, Hainan, PR China

Zu-Rui Lin
Yunnan Institute of Parasitic Diseases, Yunnan Provincial Centre of Malaria Research, Yunnan Provincial Key Laboratory of Vector-borne Diseases Control and Research, Yunnan Institute of Parasitic Diseases Innovative Team of Key Techniques for Vector Borne Disease Control and Prevention, Training Base of International Scientific Exchange and Education in Tropical Diseases for South and Southeast Asia, Puer, Yunnan, PR China

Guang-qi Liu
Department of Global Health, Peking University School of Public Health; Institute for Global Health, Peking University, Beijing, PR China

Hui Liu
Yunnan Institute of Parasitic Diseases, Yunnan Provincial Centre of Malaria Research, Yunnan Provincial Key Laboratory of Vector-borne Diseases Control and Research, Yunnan Institute of Parasitic Diseases Innovative Team of Key Techniques for Vector Borne Disease Control and Prevention, Training Base of International Scientific Exchange and Education in Tropical Diseases for South and Southeast Asia, Puer, Yunnan, PR China

Yaobao Liu
Key Laboratory of National Health Commission (NHC) on Parasitic Disease Control and Prevention, Jiangsu Provincial Key Laboratory on Parasite and Vector Control Technology, Jiangsu Institute of Parasitic Diseases, Wuxi, Jiangsu, PR China

Ying Liu
Henan Center for Disease Control and Prevention, Zhengzhou, Henan, PR China

Yong Liu
Tunchang County Center for Disease Control & Prevention, Tunchang, Yunnan, PR China

Zi-Jian Liu
Anhui Provincial Center for Disease Control and Prevention, Anhui, PR China

De-Ling Lu
Henan Center for Disease Control and Prevention, Zhengzhou, Henan, PR China

Guangyu Lu
School of Public Health, Medical College of Yangzhou University, Yangzhou University, Yangzhou, Jiangsu, PR China

Xue-Chun Lu
Anhui Provincial Center for Disease Control and Prevention, Anhui, PR China

Xiao-Feng Lv
Anhui Provincial Center for Disease Control and Prevention, Anhui, PR China

Ji-yan Maa
Department of Global Health, Peking University School of Public Health; Institute for Global Health, Peking University, Beijing, PR China

Feng Meng
Hainan Provincial Center for Disease Control & Prevention, Haikou, Hainan, PR China

Dan Qian
Henan Center for Disease Control and Prevention, Zhengzhou, Henan, PR China

Yi-nuo Sun
Department of Global Health, Peking University School of Public Health; Institute for Global Health, Peking University, Beijing, PR China

Marcel Tanner
Swiss Tropical and Public Health Institute; University of Basel, Basel, Switzerland

Dan Wang
Henan Center for Disease Control and Prevention, Zhengzhou, Henan, PR China

Guangze Wang
Hainan Provincial Center for Disease Control & Prevention, Haikou, Hainan, PR China

Guoyi Wang
Qiongzhong County Center for Disease Control & Prevention, Qiongzhong, Hainan, PR China

Jian Wang
Baisha County Center for Disease Control & Prevention, Baisha, Hainan, PR China

Jian-Jun Wang
Anhui Provincial Center for Disease Control and Prevention, Anhui, PR China

Shanqing Wang
Hainan Provincial Center for Disease Control & Prevention, Haikou, Hainan, PR China

Shu-Qi Wang
Anhui Provincial Center for Disease Control and Prevention, Anhui, PR China

Weiming Wang
Key Laboratory of National Health Commission (NHC) on Parasitic Disease Control and Prevention, Jiangsu Provincial Key Laboratory on Parasite and Vector Control Technology, Jiangsu Institute of Parasitic Diseases, Wuxi, Jiangsu, PR China

Chun Wei
Yunnan Institute of Parasitic Diseases, Yunnan Provincial Centre of Malaria Research, Yunnan Provincial Key Laboratory of Vector-borne Diseases Control and Research, Yunnan Institute of Parasitic Diseases Innovative Team of Key Techniques for Vector Borne Disease Control and Prevention, Training Base of International Scientific Exchange and Education in Tropical Diseases for South and Southeast Asia, Puer, Yunnan, PR China

Xiaodan Wen
Danzhou City Center for Disease Control & Prevention, Danzhou, Hainan, PR China

Yan Xie
Department of Global Health, Peking University School of Public Health; Institute for Global Health, Peking University, Beijing, PR China

Huanzhi Xu
Wuzhishan City Center for Disease Control & Prevention, Wuzhishan, Hainan, PR China

Jian-wei Xu
Yunnan Institute of Parasitic Diseases, Yunnan Provincial Centre of Malaria Research, Yunnan Provincial Key Laboratory of Vector-borne Diseases Control and Research, Yunnan Institute of Parasitic Diseases Innovative Team of Key Techniques for Vector Borne Disease Control and Prevention, Training Base of International Scientific Exchange and Education in Tropical Diseases for South and Southeast Asia, Puer, Yunnan, PR China

Xian Xu
Anhui Provincial Center for Disease Control and Prevention, Anhui, PR China

Bing Yang
Hainan Provincial Center for Disease Control & Prevention, Haikou, Hainan, PR China

Cheng-Yun Yang
Henan Center for Disease Control and Prevention, Zhengzhou, Henan, PR China

Mengmeng Yang
Key Laboratory of National Health Commission (NHC) on Parasitic Disease Control and Prevention, Jiangsu Provincial Key Laboratory on Parasite and Vector Control Technology, Jiangsu Institute of Parasitic Diseases, Wuxi, Jiangsu, PR China

Rongshen Ye
Baoying County Center for Disease Control & Prevention, Baoying, Jiangsu, PR China

Jian-Hai Yin
National Institute of Parasitic Diseases, Chinese Center for Disease Control and Prevention (Chinese Center for Tropical Diseases Research), NHC Key Laboratory of Parasite and Vector Biology, WHO Collaborating Center for Tropical Diseases, National Center for International Research on Tropical Diseases, Shanghai, PR China

Wen Zeng
Hainan Provincial Center for Disease Control & Prevention, Haikou, Hainan, PR China

Datian Zhan
Lingshui County Center for Disease Control & Prevention, Lingshui, Hainan, PR China

Cang-Lin Zhang
Yunnan Institute of Parasitic Diseases, Yunnan Provincial Centre of Malaria Research, Yunnan Provincial Key Laboratory of Vector-borne Diseases Control and Research, Yunnan Institute of Parasitic Diseases Innovative Team of Key Techniques for Vector Borne Disease Control and Prevention, Training Base of International Scientific Exchange and Education in Tropical Diseases for South and Southeast Asia, Puer, Yunnan, PR China

Hong-Wei Zhang
Henan Center for Disease Control and Prevention, Zhengzhou, Henan, PR China

Kai-xuan Zhang
Department of Global Health, Peking University School of Public Health; Institute for Global Health, Peking University, Beijing, PR China

Tao Zhang
Anhui Provincial Center for Disease Control and Prevention, Anhui, PR China

Ji Zhen
Dongfang City Center for Disease Control & Prevention, Dongfang, Hainan, PR China

Zaichun Zheng
Changjiang County Center for Disease Control & Prevention, Changjiang, Hainan, PR China

Hong-Ning Zhou
Yunnan Institute of Parasitic Diseases, Yunnan Provincial Centre of Malaria Research, Yunnan Provincial Key Laboratory of Vector-borne Diseases Control and Research, Yunnan Institute of Parasitic Diseases Innovative Team of Key Techniques for Vector Borne Disease Control and Prevention, Training Base of International Scientific Exchange and Education in Tropical Diseases for South and Southeast Asia, Puer, Yunnan, PR China

Huayun Zhou
Key Laboratory of National Health Commission (NHC) on Parasitic Disease Control and Prevention, Jiangsu Provincial Key Laboratory on Parasite and Vector Control Technology, Jiangsu Institute of Parasitic Diseases, Wuxi, Jiangsu, PR China

Rui-min Zhou
Henan Center for Disease Control and Prevention, Zhengzhou, Henan, PR China

Xiao-Nong Zhou
National Institute of Parasitic Diseases, Chinese Center for Disease Control and Prevention (Chinese Center for Tropical Diseases Research), NHC Key Laboratory of Parasite and Vector Biology, WHO Collaborating Center for Tropical Diseases, National Center for International Research on Tropical Diseases; School of Global Health, Chinese Center for Tropical Diseases Research, Shanghai Jiao Tong University School of Medicine, Shanghai, PR China

Yao-Wu Zhou
Yunnan Institute of Parasitic Diseases, Yunnan Provincial Centre of Malaria Research, Yunnan Provincial Key Laboratory of Vector-borne Diseases Control and Research, Yunnan Institute of Parasitic Diseases Innovative Team of Key Techniques for Vector Borne Disease Control and Prevention, Training Base of International Scientific Exchange and Education in Tropical Diseases for South and Southeast Asia, Puer, Yunnan, PR China

Guoding Zhu
Key Laboratory of National Health Commission (NHC) on Parasitic Disease Control and Prevention, Jiangsu Provincial Key Laboratory on Parasite and Vector Control Technology, Jiangsu Institute of Parasitic Diseases, Wuxi; Center for Global Health, School of Public Health, Nanjing Medical University, Nanjing, Jiangsu, PR China

A malaria-free China: global importance and key experience

Jian-Hai Yin[a], Christian Lengeler[b,c], Marcel Tanner[b,c], and Xiao-Nong Zhou[a,d]

[a]National Institute of Parasitic Diseases, Chinese Center for Disease Control and Prevention (Chinese Center for Tropical Diseases Research), NHC Key Laboratory of Parasite and Vector Biology, WHO Collaborating Centre for Tropical Diseases, National Center for International Research on Tropical Diseases, Shanghai, PR China

[b]Swiss Tropical and Public Health Institute, Basel, Switzerland

[c]University of Basel, Basel, Switzerland

[d]School of Global Health, Chinese Center for Tropical Diseases Research, Shanghai Jiao Tong University School of Medicine, Shanghai, PR China

Abstract

Malaria has a worldwide distribution and is the world's deadliest mosquito-borne disease. The goal of malaria elimination is also reflected in the United Nations Sustainable Development Goals and the Global Technical Strategy for Malaria 2016–2030 issued by the World Health Organization (WHO). China succeeded in its malaria elimination programme after being certified as malaria-free by the WHO on 30 June 2021. Therefore, we document some of the key lessons learnt in the course of the malaria elimination effort in China in this special volume, showing how different strategies made elimination feasible in different subregions of China with different epidemiological and socioeconomic characteristics, in order to present strong signals to other malaria-endemic countries that malaria elimination is feasible within one generation.

Malaria, the world's deadliest mosquito-borne disease, is both a preventable and treatable disease. In 2011, the world declared its intention of eliminating malaria, and this commitment has been re-endorsed in 2017 (WHO, 2017). The goal of malaria elimination is also reflected in the United Nations Sustainable Development Goals (UN, 2015). However, as of the beginning of 2022, there were still large areas of the world, particularly on the African continent, in which high levels of malaria transmission occurred (WHO, 2021a). The Global Technical Strategy (GTS) for Malaria 2016–2030 issued by the World Health Organization (WHO) outlined the way leading to reduced morbidity and mortality rates, and a rapidly increasing number of countries being certified as malaria-free (WHO, 2015).

Documenting carefully successful examples of countries having eliminated malaria is paramount to show the feasibility of this major public health undertaking, share crucial experience and boost political support. Between

2017 and 2020, seven E-2020 member countries succeeded in reaching the goal of malaria elimination, including: Algeria, Belize, Cabo Verde, China, El Salvador, the Islamic Republic of Iran and Malaysia (WHO, 2021b). In this special volume of *Advances in Parasitology*, we document some of the key lessons learnt in the course of the malaria elimination effort in China, one of the E-2020 member countries and the world's most populous country. China succeeded in lowering its malaria burden from 30 million cases per year in the 1940s to zero indigenous cases in 2017. It was certified as malaria-free by WHO on 30 June 2021 (WHO, 2021c). This achievement does send strong signals to other malaria-endemic countries that even in large and highly populated countries, with a great diversity of malaria transmission socioecosystems, malaria elimination is feasible within one generation. Although the malaria elimination process is different in each country, because of different ecologies, epidemiology, health system context and general socioeconomic circumstances, the key to success bears similarities in all settings (Zhou, 2021). Firstly, and most importantly, a strong and sustained political commitment, allowing the implementation of resources and actions until the very end of the elimination process. Secondly, a strong primary healthcare system with universal access to prevention and treatment for all risk groups, especially for vulnerable populations living in remote or hard-to-reach areas. Thirdly, and especially in the end phase, a robust surveillance and response system for rapid detection of malaria transmission and infection followed by investigation and public health response packages tailored to the situation, which will interrupt transmission and thus eliminate transmission pockets. Fourthly, quality-assured sensitive and specific diagnostics under the supervision of a network of high-quality reference laboratories. And fifthly, pragmatic multisectoral collaborations and effective cross-border collaborations along international borders, to prevent malaria from re-establishing itself (WHO, 2021b).

China went through a phase of progressive control with its national malaria control programme in 1950–2009, although several subphases presented in the long-term course of the control phase, while the national malaria elimination programme was initiated in 2010 (Feng et al., 2018; Yin et al., 2014). Hence, China went through a control phase, followed by an elimination phase, and it has now entered the postelimination phase. Its successes were based on continuously updated and adapted technical measures and strategies, particularly the 1-3-7 surveillance and response approach (Cao et al., 2014; Zhou et al., 2015), the establishment of the 'National Information Management System for Parasitic Disease Control and Prevention' and a national malaria diagnostic reference laboratory network. The tools and strategies were based on and tailored to the realities on the ground, and complemented by innovative research and implementation science. Moreover, the overall socioeconomic developments across the country, through intensive implementation of poverty alleviation projects, international cooperation, as well as active community involvement in the form of patriotic public health campaigns, were major determinants, and all of these contributed to the success of malaria elimination.

In the current postelimination phase, China's focus is preventing the reintroduction of malaria from neighbouring countries in Asia as well as returning labourers from African countries. At the same time, China also carefully documented the lessons learnt from its successful experience for the benefit of other malaria-endemic countries (Chen et al., 2021). To this end, the National Institute of Parasitic Diseases of the Chinese Center for Disease Control and Prevention (China CDC) (Xiao et al., 2020)—with support from the Bill and Melinda Gates Foundation—coordinated a group of more than 30 experts to review and document the lessons learnt from the Chinese malaria elimination experience from practices and evidence. These case studies are published in the present special volume of *Accomplishment of Malaria Elimination in the People's Republic of China*. The volume documents how different strategies made elimination feasible in different subregions of China with different epidemiological and socioeconomic characteristics. It includes careful description and analyses of

(i) the 1-3-7 surveillance and response approach in Jiangsu Province (Cao et al., 2022),
(ii) malaria control and elimination along the border areas in Yunnan Province (Liu et al., 2022a),
(iii) malaria response focused on forest goers in the mountainous areas in Hainan island (Li et al., 2022),
(iv) focal mass drug administration for *Plasmodium vivax* control in Anhui Province (Xu et al., 2022), and
(v) malaria re-emergence response in Henan Province (Liu et al., 2022b).

In addition to these examples of best practices, the volume also documents the key contributions of Chinese scientists to the global malaria control and elimination effort, such as the discovery of artemisinin in China which led to the Nobel Prize being awarded to Dr Tu Youyou in 2015 (Liu et al., 2022c). Another example was that Chinese experiences on 1-3-7 surveillance and response approach, reported in this special issue, has been adapted towards a 1,7-malaria reactive community-based testing and response (1, 7-mRCTR) approach adequate for Coastal Tanzania. The coherent implementation of the 1, 7-mRCTR approach reduced malaria incidence by 80% within 3 years (Mlacha et al., 2020; Wang et al., 2019).

We hope that the experiences published in this special volume will further support the global malaria elimination programme, especially the E-2025 initiative (WHO, 2021b). The Chinese experience combined with successful elimination experience in other countries shows how the current GTS (WHO, 2015) provides the technical guidance to move from elimination towards eradication in the generations to come, as considered scientifically and politically feasible in the respective report of the Strategic Advisory Group of WHO in 2019 (WHO, 2019). Sharing and comparing the wealth of operational and strategic experience globally across systems and cultures will benefit all individuals still suffering from the scourge of malaria.

References

Cao, J., Sturrock, H.J.W., Cotter, C., Zhou, S., Zhou, H., Liu, Y., Tang, L., Gosling, R.D., Feachem, R.G.A., Gao, Q., 2014. Communicating and monitoring surveillance and response activities for malaria elimination China's "1-3-7" strategy. PLoS Med. 11, e1001642.

Cao, Y., Lu, G., Zhou, H., Wang, W., Liu, Y., Yang, M., Liang, C., Zhu, G., Cao, J., 2022. Case-based malaria surveillance and response: implementation of 1-3-7 approach in Jiangsu Province, China. Adv. Parasitol. 116, 1–31.

Chen, J.H., Fen, J., Zhou, X.N., 2021. From 30 million to zero malaria cases in China: lessons learned for China-Africa collaboration in malaria elimination. Infect. Dis. Poverty 10 (1), 51.

Feng, J., Zhang, L., Huang, F., Yin, J.H., Tu, H., Xia, Z.G., Zhou, S.S., Xiao, N., Zhou, X.N., 2018. Ready for malaria elimination: zero indigenous case reported in the People's Republic of China. Malar. J. 17 (1), 315.

Li,Y., Wang, S., Hu,X., Huang,Y., Chen, R., Lin, M., Xu, H., Ye, R., Zhan, D., Huang, S., Zhen, J., Wen, X., Wang, G., Liu, Y., Li, H., Zheng, Z., Wang, J., Zeng, W., Meng, F., Huang, X., Wang, G., Yang, B.,Chen, Y., 2022. Surveillance and response systems driving malaria elimination in the mountain areas of Hainan Province. Adv. Parasitol. 116, 69–113.

Liu, H., Zhou,Y.-W., Deng, Y., Lin, Z.-R., Zhang, C.-L., Chen,Q.-Y., Wei, C., Duan, K.-X., Zhou, H.-N., Xu, J.-w., 2022a. Historical review of malaria control and elimination in the border areas of China: a case study of Yunnan Province. Adv. Parasitol. 116, 33–67.

Liu, Y., He, Z.-Q., Wang, D., Hu, Y.-B., Qian, D., Yang, C.-Y., Zhou, R.-m., Li, S.-H., Lu, D.-L., Zhang, H.-W., 2022b. One Health approach to improve the malaria elimination programme in Henan Province. Adv. Parasitol. 116, 153–186.

Liu, G.-q., Xie, Y., Sun, Y.-n., Zhang, K.-x., Maa, J.-y., Huang, Y.-m., 2022c. Research and development of traditional medicines in low- and middle-income countries: a case study of artemisinin discovery in China. Adv. Parasitol. 116, 187–209.

Mlacha, Y.P., Wang, D., Chaki, P.P., Gavana, T., Zhou, Z., Michael, M.G., Khatib, R., Chila, G., Msuya, H.M., Chaki, E., et al., 2020. Effectiveness of the innovative 1,7-malaria reactive community-based testing and response (1,7-mRCTR) approach on malaria burden reduction in Southeastern Tanzania. Malar. J. 19 (1), 292.

UN, 2015. Transforming Our World: The 2030 Agenda for Sustainable Development. United Nations, New York, NY.

Wang, D., Chaki, P., Mlacha, Y., Gavana, T., Michael, M.G., Khatibu, R., Feng, J., Zhou, Z.B., Lin, K.M., Xia, S., et al., 2019. Application of community-based and integrated strategy to reduce malaria disease burden in southern Tanzania: the study protocol of China-UK-Tanzania pilot project on malaria control. Infect. Dis. Poverty 8 (1), 4.

WHO, 2015. Global Technical Strategy for Malaria 2016–2030. WHO Press, Geneva, Switzerland.
WHO, 2017. A Framework for Malaria Elimination. WHO Press, Geneva, Switzerland.
WHO, 2019. Malaria Eradication: Benefits, Future Scenarios and Feasibility. Executive Summary, WHO Strategic Advisory Group on Malaria Eradication. World Health Organization, Geneva, Switzerland. (WHO/CDS/GMP/2019.10). License: CC BY-NC-SA 3.0 IGO.
WHO, 2021a. World Malaria Report 2021. WHO Press, Geneva, Switzerland.
WHO, 2021b. Zeroing in on Malaria Elimination: Final Report of the E-2020 Initiative. WHO Press, Geneva, Switzerland.
WHO, 2021c. From 30 Million Cases to Zero: China Is Certified Malaria-Free by WHO. https://www.who.int/news/item/30-06-2021-from-30-million-cases-to-zero-china-is-certified-malaria-free-by-who. (accessed 6 February 2022).
Xiao, N., Li, S.Z., Qian, M.B., Xia, Z.G., Yu, Q., Liu, Q., Lv, S., Zhou, X.N., 2020. Contribution of NIPD-CTDR to the parasitic diseases control and elimination in China: memory of the 70th anniversary for NIPD-CTDR. Adv. Parasitol. 110, 401–427.
Xu, X., Wang, J.-J., Jiang, J.-J., Zhang, T., Lv, X.-F., Wang, S.-Q., Liu, Z.-J., Li, W.-D., Lu, X.-C., 2022. Mass drug administration in response to vivax malaria resurgence in Anhui Province of Huanghuai Plain, China. Adv. Parasitol. 116, 115–152.
Yin, J.H., Zhou, S.S., Xia, Z.G., Wang, R.B., Qian, Y.J., Yang, W.Z., Zhou, X.N., 2014. Historical patterns of malaria transmission in China. Adv. Parasitol. 86, 1–19.
Zhou, X.N., 2021. China declared malaria-free: a milestone in the world malaria eradication and Chinese public health. Infect. Dis. Poverty 10 (1), 98.
Zhou, S.S., Zhang, S.S., Zhang, L., Rietveld, A.E.C., Ramsay, A.R., Zachariah, R., Bissell, K., Bergh, R.V.D., Xia, Z.G., Zhou, X.N., Cibulskis, R.E., 2015. China's 1-3-7 surveillance and response strategy for malaria elimination: is case reporting, investigation and foci response happening according to plan? Infect. Dis. Poverty 4, 55.

CHAPTER ONE

Case-based malaria surveillance and response: implementation of 1-3-7 approach in Jiangsu Province, China

Yuanyuan Cao[a,†], Guangyu Lu[b,†], Huayun Zhou[a], Weiming Wang[a], Yaobao Liu[a], Mengmeng Yang[a], Cheng Liang[a], Guoding Zhu[a,c,*], and Jun Cao[a,c,*]

[a]Key Laboratory of National Health Commission (NHC) on Parasitic Disease Control and Prevention, Jiangsu Provincial Key Laboratory on Parasite and Vector Control Technology, Jiangsu Institute of Parasitic Diseases, Wuxi, Jiangsu, PR China
[b]School of Public Health, Medical College of Yangzhou University, Yangzhou University, Yangzhou, Jiangsu, PR China
[c]Center for Global Health, School of Public Health, Nanjing Medical University, Nanjing, Jiangsu, PR China
*Corresponding authors: e-mail address: jipdzhu@hotmail.com; caojuncn@hotmail.com

Contents

1. Introduction 2
2. Background 3
   2.1 Geography, population and health system of Jiangsu Province 3
   2.2 Malaria epidemic situation in Jiangsu Province 4
   2.3 Malaria control phase in Jiangsu Province 5
   2.4 Malaria elimination phase in Jiangsu Province 8
3. Needs of intensive malaria surveillance and response approach 10
   3.1 Surveillance system for malaria elimination globally 10
   3.2 Needs of intensive malaria surveillance and response approach in China 11
   3.3 Introduction of malaria 1-3-7 surveillance and response approach 13
4. Implementation of malaria 1-3-7 surveillance and response approach in Jiangsu Province 15
   4.1 Case reporting within 1 day 16
   4.2 Case confirmation and classification within 3 days 17
   4.3 Focus investigation and action within 7 days 18
5. Challenges for implementing malaria 1-3-7 approach in Jiangsu Province 20
   5.1 The sensitivity of the malaria surveillance system needs to be improved 20
   5.2 Innovative strategies in the management of mobile and migrant populations need to be implemented 21

† Yuanyuan Cao and Guangyu Lu contributed equally to this work.

Advances in Parasitology, Volume 116
ISSN 0065-308X
https://doi.org/10.1016/bs.apar.2022.04.003

5.3 The delayed presentation of malaria patients to healthcare needs to be intervened 22
5.4 The malaria surveillance and response system needs to be sustained 22
6. Lessons learned from implementing malaria 1-3-7 approach in Jiangsu Province 23
6.1 A well-established communicable disease reporting system is essential 23
6.2 Strengthening of surveillance for malaria case detection by optimizing the malaria blood testing network 24
6.3 Strengthening malaria diagnostic capacity at primary health facilitates 24
6.4 Establishment of quality control system for malaria diagnosis 25
6.5 Multisectoral coordination mechanism and management of migrant population 26
6.6 Conducting operational research and supervision to facilitate the implementation of the 1-3-7 approach 27
6.7 International exchange and cooperation 27
7. Conclusions 28
Acknowledgements 28
References 28

Abstract

Following initiation of China's National Malaria Elimination Action Plan (NMEAP) in 2010, China's 1-3-7 surveillance and response approach was developed and rolled out in China to facilitate the malaria control programme and accelerate the progress of malaria elimination. Innovative strategies and interventions have been developed and implemented in Jiangsu Province to facilitate case-based malaria surveillance and response. A total of 9879 malaria cases were reported in Jiangsu Province from 2001 to 2020. Since 2012, no indigenous malaria cases have been reported in Jiangsu Province. However, in recent years, there has been a substantial increase of imported cases from abroad. To continue improving the malaria surveillance and response system, Jiangsu Province has conducted population-based health education to improve the healthcare seeking behaviour of malaria patients, strengthened the capacity of health facilities to improve the performance of malaria diagnosis and treatment, and strengthened health workforce capacity to improve the implementation of 1-3-7 approach. Continually improving surveillance and response system can play a critical role in the early detection and rapid response of individual malaria cases and prevent the re-establishment of malaria.

1. Introduction

Malaria was once one of major tropical diseases that exerted a great burden on people's health, as well as the social and economic development in the People's Republic of China (P.R. China), particularly in the period from 1950 to 1970s, when annual malaria cases numbered mostly around several millions. The government of P.R. China has paid great efforts to malaria control during the last seven decades. On June 30, 2021, China was officially certified as malaria-free by WHO and is the first country in the WHO Western Pacific Region to be awarded a malaria-free certification in more than three decades (WHO, 2021).

In malaria elimination programmes, surveillance and response system should be highly vigilant and effective to block any transmission. One of China's experiences helping to reach this milestone, the 1-3-7 surveillance and response approach was implemented in China in early 2012 (Cao et al., 2014). The 1-3-7 approach refers to report malaria cases within 1 day, confirm and investigate the reported case within 3 days, and then take appropriate focus/foci disposition to prevent further transmission within 7 days. The main objective of this chapter is to introduce the initialization, working scheme, and implementation of the China's 1-3-7 approach in Jiangsu Province. We also summarized the potential challenges that need to be addressed in implementing the China's 1-3-7 approach in order to prevent malaria re-establishment in China. In additional, we synthesized the lessons learned from the 1-3-7 approach, which will benefit the development and implementation of adapted malaria surveillance and response approaches in other malaria endemic countries.

2. Background

2.1 Geography, population and health system of Jiangsu Province

Jiangsu Province is situated in the central part of the eastern coastal area of China, where located in the downstream of Yangtze River and Huaihe River, borders the Yellow Sea in the east, Shandong Province in the north, Anhui Province in the west, and Shanghai City and Zhejiang Province in the southeast (Fig. 1). Jiangsu Province is located at north latitude 30° 45′N-35°20′N and east longitude 116°18′–121°57′. Jiangsu Province covers an area of 107,200 km^2 with 13 cities and a population of 80.293 million in 2017. The 13 prefectures in Jiangsu Province were divided into three groups: the most economically developed southern zone (including Nanjing, Zhenjiang, Suzhou, Wuxi and Changzhou), the moderately developed middle zone (including Yangzhou, Taizhou and Nantong) and the less economically active northern zone (including Xuzhou, Lianyungang, Suqian, Huai'an, and Yancheng). The province is located in a transition belt from a subtropical to temperate zone, with an annual temperature ranged between

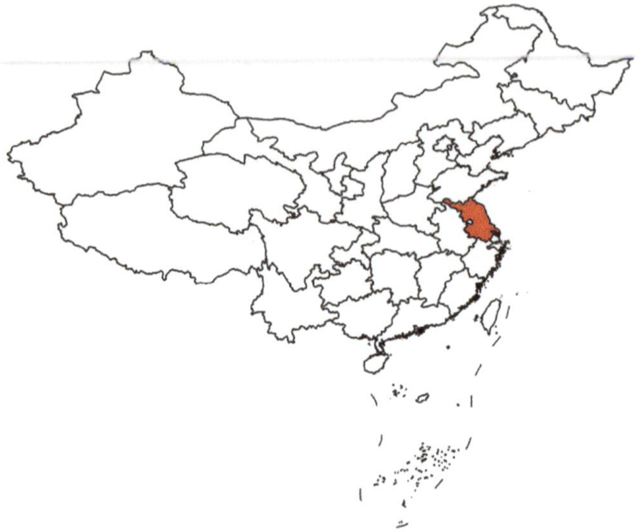

Fig. 1 Geographical location of Jiangsu Province in China.

13 and 16 °C and moderate rainfall of average annual precipitation 1528.5 mm. It is the only province in China that is home to important seas, rivers and lakes, has numerous lakes and a dense network of waterways, with an overall water area accounting for 16.9% of its territory (Jiangsu Provincial People's Government, 2021). The climate and environment is suitable for the breeding of Anopheles, including *Anopheles sinensis* and *Anopheles anthropophagus.*

Jiangsu's health system is composed of hospitals, centres for disease control and prevention (CDCs), as well as microscopy stations affiliated with them at all levels. In 2016, there were 32,080 health institutions in total, including 1033 provincial, prefectural and county general hospitals, 3701 grassroots health centres and community health service centres, 117 provincial municipal and county CDCs across Jiangsu Province. Moreover, there were estimated 517,065 medical and health personnel at all levels (Jiangsu Commission of Health, 2016).

2.2 Malaria epidemic situation in Jiangsu Province

Historically, Jiangsu Province was a highly malaria endemic area. The main vectors of malaria in Jiangsu Province are *An. sinensis* and *An. anthropophagus.* Of these, *An. sinensis* is the dominant malaria-transmitting vector in Jiangsu Province, and the climate and environment is suitable for the breeding of *Anopheles* mosquitoes (Zhu et al., 2014). The major indigenous parasite species in Jiangsu Province is *Plasmodium vivax*. Two major outbreaks of malaria in Jiangsu Province occurred in the year of 1960 and 1971. In Jiangsu Province, the annual malaria incidence rate during the 1960s was 24.95%, which caused a serious threat to public health and hindered social and economic development. In the later 1980s, the incidence of malaria deceased to less than 1/10,000 with the implementation of comprehensive control measures, and later reduced to less than 1/100,000 in 1993. While, the malaria epidemic was unstable in 1990s. In 1997, there was a small-scale outbreak in Xuyi County, the area with *An. sinensis* and *An. anthropophagus*, and the incidence of malaria increased from 0.20/10,000 in 1996 to 12.18/10,000 in 1997. There have been small-scale malaria outbreaks in Suqian and Xuzhou city, but all the malaria outbreaks were successfully suppressed. Notably, the number of malaria cases imported from abroad increased sharply since 2005. In 2010, 248 cases with malaria imported from abroad were reported in the province, and for the first time the number of cases with imported malaria from abroad exceeded the number of indigenous malaria cases (Zhou et al., 2012). In the following years, the number of indigenous cases further declined, while the number of cases with imported malaria from abroad has remained at a high level (Zhou et al., 2009a,b). After decades-long efforts, the last indigenous case in Jiangsu was reported in 2011. Therefore, cases with imported malaria have been become a major concern in the province (Fig. 2).

2.3 Malaria control phase in Jiangsu Province

From the foundation of P.R. China in 1949 to the launch of China's National Malaria Elimination Action Plan (NMEAP) in 2010, the malaria transmission and control in Jiangsu Province can be described into four stages: (1) establishing the health system for diseases prevention and control (1951–1959), (2) controlling malaria outbreaks (1960–1979), (3) shrinking malaria burden with comprehensive control measures (1980–1999), and (4) transiting from malaria control to elimination (2000–2009).

(1) Stage I: establishing the health system for diseases prevention and control (1951–1959)

In 1950, the Jiangsu Institute of Parasitic Diseases (JIPD) was firstly established at the provincial level. JIPD is responsible for training professionals, conducting epidemiological investigations, and carrying out researches on parasitic diseases, mainly concentrated in malaria and schistosomiasis in particular. Following this initiative, health promotion and epidemic prevention

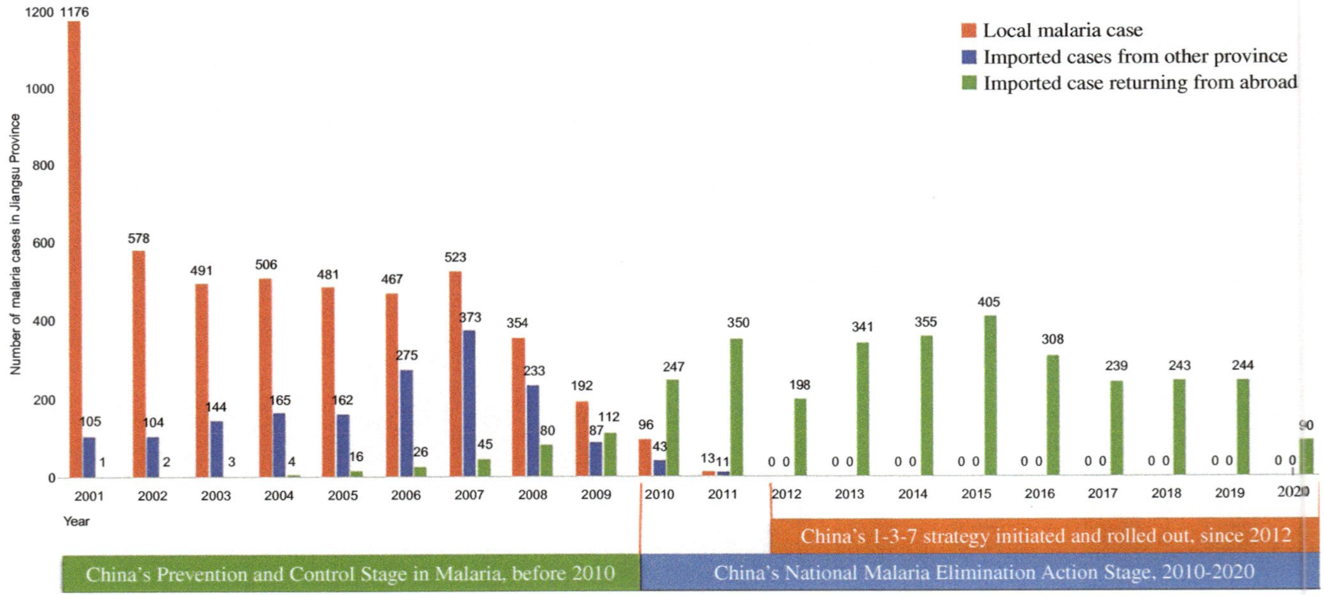

Fig. 2 Reported number of malaria cases from 2001 to 2020 in Jiangsu Province.

stations (or named as malaria control stations) were established at different administrative levels in the province. They are mainly responsible for the prevention and control of local highly endemic parasitic diseases, e.g., malaria and schistosomiasis. In 1959, reducing the mortality and morbidity of malaria has been proposed as a primary task. However, due to inadequate reporting capacity and health infrastructure, malaria remained to be one of the most highly endemic infectious diseases in Jiangsu Province.

(2) Stage II: controlling malaria outbreaks (1960–1979)

In 1960, mainly affected by natural disasters, Jiangsu Province experienced the first large scale malaria outbreak since the foundation of the P.R. China in 1949. In order to effectively control malaria outbreaks, large-scale malaria control activities at the population level were carried out in Jiangsu Province. It mainly included providing anti-relapse treatment for patients with *vivax* malaria history and who were in resting stage; providing prophylactic medication in malaria highly endemic areas during malaria transmission seasons and reducing mosquito breeding sites. The malaria outbreaks have been controlled and the incidence of malaria was significantly reduced through these comprehensive measures (Zhou et al., 2009a,b). However, in 1973, anti-malarial activities have been interrupted and another large scale *vivax* malaria outbreak occurred. In order to control this outbreak, Jiangsu Province started to provide anti-relapse treatment to whole population in malaria resting stage, provide prophylactic medication to whole population during malaria transmission season and re-treat patients including children with malaria history during malaria transmission season in 46 epidemic cities/counties regularly. Mass drug administration (MDA) with pyrimethamine and primaquine was performed on a large scale involving millions of people to treat potential reservoirs of *P. vivax* blood and liver stage infection before the start of the malaria transmission season (Hsiang et al., 2013). During this period, *P. falciparum* had nearly been eliminated from Jiangsu Province, with only some 140 annual cases reported (Hsiang et al., 2013). Since 1974, Jiangsu Province participated in the "Joint Malaria Control and Prevention in Central Five Provinces" programme (Jiangsu, Shandong, Henan, Anhui and Hubei provinces). The five provinces joint initiative on anti-malaria largely promoted the effective implementation of malaria prevention and control measures in Central China (Shang et al., 2006).

(3) Stage III: shrinking malaria burden with comprehensive control measures (1980–1999)

Starting from 1979, Jiangsu Province initialized comprehensive control measures including vector control, prophylactic medication to whole population in highly endemic areas during malaria-transmitted seasons, and in provision of anti-relapse treatment to patients with *vivax* malaria, in resting stage, and blood testing and treatment to fever patients. The main vector control measures included the extensively indoor residual spraying of DDT and administration of deltamethrin-treated mosquito nets. In 1980, Jiangsu Province started to build outpatient malaria microscopy stations mainly based on the township hospitals' labs. By 1984, a network consisted of more than 2000 outpatient microscopy stations at provincial, prefectural, county and townships levels had been built in Jiangsu. During 1974–1988, a total of 23,673,408 fever patients were examined through microscopy across Jiangsu Province. From 1974 to 1988, 6,258,284 person-times were treated for patients with malaria, 144,978,238 person-times were treated for patients with malaria history in the resting stage, and 278,141,117 person-times have been taken by prophylactic medication in Jiangsu Province. The annual incidence of malaria dropped from 2495/10,000 in 1960 to 0.64/10,000 in 1988 (Zhou et al., 2009a,b). By 1988, no indigenous *P. falciparum* cases had been reported in Jiangsu Province.

(4) Stage IV: transiting from malaria control to elimination (1990–2009) Under the implementation of comprehensive malaria prevention and control measures, an ever-strengthening public health system, a strong political commitment and the financial support of Global Fund to fight AIDS, Tuberculosis and Malaria, malaria burden was largely reduced. In Jiangsu Province, the annual number of cases had fallen from 2906 in 1990 to 389 in 2009 and the incidence of malaria dropped from 0.42/10,000 in 1989 to 0.05/10,000 in 2009. In Jiangsu Province, from 1989 to 2009, 19,020,208 patients with fevers received blood tests of plasmodium. A total of 20,538 patients with malaria, 1,733,505 patients with malaria history and in malaria resting stage were treated, and 2,764,476 people received prophylactic medication during malaria-transmitted seasons. Sporadic malaria outbreaks occurred during this period and all were effectively controlled.

2.4 Malaria elimination phase in Jiangsu Province

In September 2010, in accordance with the overall requirements on NMEAP (2010–2020), Jiangsu Provincial People's Government issued the Jiangsu Malaria Elimination Action Plan (2010–2020) and the malaria elimination in Jiangsu Province started from then on (Jiangsu Provincial People's Government, 2010).

Since the launch of malaria elimination action plan, Jiangsu Province has showed a strong political commitment to eliminating malaria in the province. The Jiangsu Commission of Health (former Provincial Department of Health) formulated and issued *Jiangsu Malaria Elimination Work Program* every year to clarify the specific tasks and measures on malaria elimination plan. In accordance with the circumstances of Jiangsu Province, Jiangsu Institute of Parasitic Diseases (JIPD) released a series of operational guidance on malaria elimination activities, including *Jiangsu Malaria Surveillance Points Work Program*, *Jiangsu Malaria Elimination Implementation Program (2010–2012)*, *Jiangsu Usage and Management of Antimalarial Drugs Program (Trial)*, *Jiangsu Malaria Elimination Surveillance Program*, *Jiangsu Mosquito Vector Monitoring Program in Pilot Regions*, and *Jiangsu Pilot Implementation Program on the Standardized Usage of Malaria Rapid Diagnose Test.*

With the start of malaria elimination programme nationwide, Jiangsu Province has shifted the focus of the programme from reducing the number of malaria cases and deaths at population level to testing each individual malaria case and tracing it to its geographic origin to find the source of infection and contain its spread. Following the four-catalogue classification of transmission settings based on malaria transmission risk and incidence at county level, counties in Jiangsu Province were also categorized into four types (National Health Commission of China, 2010). According to the classification, 82 counties/districts in Jiangsu Province have been classified into type 2 and other 31 counties have been classified into type 3. In type 2 counties, comprehensive anti-malaria measures were taken with the aim to clear malaria infectious source and interrupt malaria transmission. In type 3 counties, strengthening malaria surveillance capacity and management of cases with imported malaria were emphasized to prevent any secondary infections.

Since malaria should also be considered in any person with fever of unknown origin regardless of travel history, malaria diagnostic capacity was strengthened and blood testing was increased for "three fevers" patients (fevers patients with malaria, with suspected malaria, and with fever of unknown reason). From 2011 to 2020, malaria blood tests for 3,637,562 "three fevers" patients were carried out in the medical facilities at all levels in Jiangsu Province, and 2797 positive for *plasmodium* species were found. Moreover, since 2012, the provincial malaria diagnosis and quality control system led by the Jiangsu Provincial Malaria Diagnosis Reference Laboratory (JMDRL) affiliated with JIPD was established, thereby improved the mechanism for case reporting, case confirmation, treatment, investigation of malaria cases. For example, from 2012 to 2020, 3052 patients' blood smears which initially reported as malaria were collected and delivered to JIPD and were re-checked by the JMDRL using microscopy and (or) nucleic acid detection (PCR), and the recheck conformity rate of the blood smears was 86.78%.

From 2011 to 2020, a total of 2797 malaria cases were reported in Jiangsu Province, of which 2769 cases were imported from abroad, accounting for 98.99% of the total number of the reported cases with malaria. During this decade, four transfused infection cases were reported (4/2797, 0.15%) (Zhang et al., 2020). There were 13 cases of local infection (13/2797, 0.47%) and 11 malaria cases (11/2797, 0.39%) originated from other provinces in China. The reported number of death in 2011, 2012 and 2014 were 3, 1 and 2 respectively, and the mortality rate was 0.21% during this period. Among the 2797 malaria cases, 2762 are diagnosed in the laboratory and 35 are diagnosed via clinical symptoms. The last indigenous case in Jiangsu Province were reported in the year 2011 (Zhou et al., 2013), who was infected with *P. vivax* and reported by Tianganghu Township Health Center, Sihong County of Suqian ctiy on September 15, 2011. In 2017, all cities and counties/districts in the province had been evaluated and reached sub-national malaria elimination assessment standards (Wang et al., 2019a,b). By 2020, no local malaria case has been reported in the Jiangsu Province for past 9 years (Wang et al., 2020).

3. Needs of intensive malaria surveillance and response approach

3.1 Surveillance system for malaria elimination globally

Surveillance is the continuous and systematic collection, analysis and interpretation of disease-specific data, and the use of that data in the planning, implementation and evaluation of public health practice (WHO, 2006). Surveillance is the backbone of disease prevention and control and is particularly critical to malaria elimination programmes, providing the disease intelligence necessary to target interventions and monitor their effectiveness. Strengthening malaria surveillance is fundamental to programme planning and implementation and is a crucial factor for accelerating progress (Moonen et al., 2010; WHO, 2015a,b, 2017).

However, there were bottlenecks in the surveillance and response strategies and key technical measures in malaria elimination stage where hindered achievement of eliminating malaria globally. Although WHO and other international research institutions have put forward some guiding advice on the strategies and measures to eliminate malaria, they are relatively difficult to operate.

In the process of malaria elimination implementation, countries are suggested to transit to surveillance systems reporting aggregated case data towards systems that facilitate rapid confirmation, investigation, and reporting of individual cases, and provide enhanced analytic methods to guide decision making related to anti-malaria interventions by WHO (WHO, 2017). After elimination has been achieved, the role of surveillance becomes a core intervention in the stage of malaria preventing re-establishment of malaria.

3.2 Needs of intensive malaria surveillance and response approach in China

In China, when moved from malaria control to malaria elimination stage, the characteristics of the malaria epidemic has been changed significantly. Local malaria cases decreased sharply in China. However, imported malaria cases overseas risen mostly originated from Sub-Saharan Africa and Southeast Asia. Zero case of local malaria was reported in China in 2017. In control stage, China focused on population-based interventions. However, during the malaria elimination stage, China should change malaria control and prevention strategy and approach into case-based sensitive surveillance and rapid response and facilitate it. New strategy and approach of malaria elimination in China shall be developed to support NMEAP. Case-based malaria surveillance and response shall play a key role during the malaria elimination stage. Through surveillance and response, we can not only find every infectious source and possible transmission focus/foci in time during elimination stage, but also provide clues and block possible transmission. After initiation of the national malaria elimination, the needs of malaria surveillance and response approach was urgently investigated in early 2012 (Cao et al., 2014). The development of the malaria surveillance and response approach has time-bound targets for case reporting, investigation, and focus/foci response activities was discussed and started to be performed at national level, in order to address the following questions and needs: how to transit from control to elimination? how to well fit the changing malaria epidemiology? how to better perform the case management with increasing number of imported malaria cases? And how to establish proper health surveillance system and infrastructure to support malaria elimination?

3.2.1 The transition of the national goal from control to elimination

The national action plan for malaria elimination in China (2010–2020) was issued by the Chinese Ministry of Health along with other 13 ministries and commissions in 2010, with the ultimate goal of the national action plan was to eliminate local transmission of malaria by 2020 (National Health Commission of the People's Republic of China, 2010). After the initialization of the elimination programme, case-based surveillance and response approach has been acknowledged as the most important components driving the whole process of the NMEAP (Feng et al., 2014). Examination of malaria parasites for all suspected cases, quality control of the examination, timely case reporting, and comprehensive case/foci investigation were emphasized.

3.2.2 The changing status on epidemiology of malaria during elimination phase

Since the launch of malaria elimination programme nationwide, continuous progress has been made through the implementation of the NMEAP. Nationwide indigenous malaria was limited to 41 counties in five provinces and 12 counties in three provinces in 2012 and 2013, respectively (Feng et al., 2015; Zhang et al., 2014). Despite an 89.8% decrease in total cases from 2008 (26,873) through 2012 (2729), the proportion of imported malaria cases has increased from 14.7% to 89.0% (Zhou et al., 2009a,b). Imported malaria cases have been reported in almost all Chinese counties since 2010, with these mainly being migrant workers returning from malaria-endemic countries (Lu et al., 2014; Zheng et al., 2013). The changing malaria epidemiology was also seen in Jiangsu Province, imported malaria cases accounted for over 70% of all malaria cases since 2010 (Zhou et al., 2012) and thus have become a major public health challenge (Zhou et al., 2016). Therefore, establishing a higher-standard case-based surveillance and response system, by which the changing epidemiology of malaria could be analysed and monitored, is important for identifying transmission foci in the province and thus guiding proper actions to prevent further transmission.

3.2.3 Better performance on case management with more imported malaria cases during elimination phase

With the rapid growth of Chinese oversea travel and increasing investment in overseas projects from China in the last decades (Liu et al., 2014), imported malaria has been increasingly reported since the launch of the NMEAP in China (Zhou et al., 2016). The imported malaria cases might reintroduce parasites and thus cause the resurgence of local transmission, where has occurred in some countries that have eliminated malaria (Cohen et al., 2012). In Jiangsu Province, a total of 2797 malaria cases were reported from 2011 to 2020, of which 2786 cases were imported. In order to cope with the increasing number of the cases with imported malaria, the reactive case detection (RACD) was considered to be the most widely adopted surveillance and response approach that targets a household or groups of households and other contacts of passively detected cases in a focus and is often deployed in combination with vector control and community education and participation (Cotter et al., 2017; Moonen et al., 2010). Therefore, China's 1-3-7 approach was developed as one of the ways to practice such a reactive surveillance and response.

3.2.4 *Well-established diseases surveillance system and infrastructure to support malaria elimination*

After severe acute respiratory syndrome (SARS) outbreak, China established the National Notifiable Infectious Disease Surveillance System and the Public Health Emergency Event Surveillance System to report disease surveillance in 2004. Clearly set out the required information and time limits for the reporting of infectious disease outbreaks and epidemics (Zhang et al., 2017). In accordance with the China infectious diseases law, malaria is listed as a notifiable disease (Category B). All malaria cases including suspected, clinically diagnosed and confirmed malaria cases must be reported by health facilities within 24h. Well-established internet-based real-time reporting system has been founded through the Chinese Information System for Disease Control and Prevention (CISDCP) (Ma et al., 2006, 2007).

With the launch of the NMEAP, the Information Management System Specific to Malaria Elimination (IMSME) and a cell phone-based short message (SMS) alert system were incorporated with CISDCP (Ma et al., 2006, 2007). Although surveillance systems for infectious diseases in China are mainly hospital based, a multi-layer administrative mechanism was adopted to enable rapid and efficient upward flow of epidemic information (Zhang and Wilson, 2012). Once a suspected, clinically diagnosed, or confirmed malaria case is reported, that CDC staff would immediately contact the reporting unit to check on the blood smear of the reported case. All information including the laboratory test and classification based on the epidemiological individual survey were required to be reported in the CISDCP system. Once confirmed, the relevant information will be reported through CISDCP and China's 1-3-7 approach would be initiated and take rapid response (Zhou et al., 2015).

3.3 Introduction of malaria 1-3-7 surveillance and response approach

Based on the principles in establishment of better surveillance and response system, malaria elimination requires intensive surveillance systems that can reliably rapidly detect and respond to individual cases. China's 1-3-7 approach was proposed, which defines targets used to guide and monitor case reporting, investigation, and response, respectively: reporting of malaria cases within 1 day, their confirmation and investigation within 3 days, and the appropriate public health response to prevent further transmission within 7 days. The 1-3-7 approach is a valuable and simple set of targets that well promoted the national malaria elimination programme with following major components (Cao et al., 2014).

1: Case reporting within 1 day. Any confirmed and suspected malaria cases by law must be reported to the web-based health information system within 24 h of diagnosis by the local health-care provider.

3: Case investigation within 3 days. All malaria cases should be confirmed and visited by the county-level China CDC, where the case is reported within 3 days, to determine where the case originated (local or imported).

7: Focus investigation and action within 7 days. The focus investigation should be conducted as soon as possible. If local transmission is possible or confirmed, targeted action to seek out other infections and reduce the chance of onward transmission is completed within 7 days by the county-level China CDC of the county where the patient resides and/or works (Fig. 3).

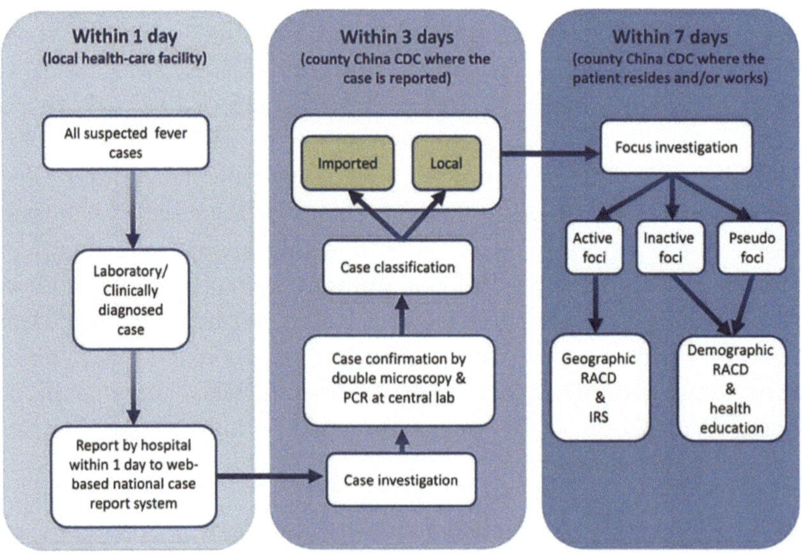

Fig. 3 Schematic of the chain of events conducted within the 1-3-7 time windows (Cao et al., 2014).

4. Implementation of malaria 1-3-7 surveillance and response approach in Jiangsu Province

From 2001 to 2020, a total of 9879 malaria cases were reported via CISDCP in Jiangsu Province. Only 13 indigenous vivax malaria were reported in 2011. Since 2012, there was no local vivax malaria cases in Jiangsu Province. Imported malaria cases were totally returned from African, Southeast Asian and South American countries, mainly originated from Equatorial Guinea (532 cases, 21.96%), Angola (526 cases, 21.71%), Nigeria (272 cases, 11.23%), Republic of Congo (138 cases, 5.693%), Cameroon (114 cases, 4.71%), accounting for 65.29% (1582 cases) from 2012 to 2020. During the 20 years, Jiangsu Province has established a malaria surveillance and response system network for malaria case finding, reporting via CISDCP within 1 day, epidemiological investigation within 3 days, and focal/foci disposal within 7 days (Fig. 4). Furthermore, in order to encourage early malaria case detection and reporting, rewards mechanism has been established when local CDC staffs reported, confirmed and disposed of malaria cases and focus/foci during malaria elimination phase. The implementation of the time-bound targets for case reporting, case investigation and foci response in Jiangsu Province was evaluated annually.

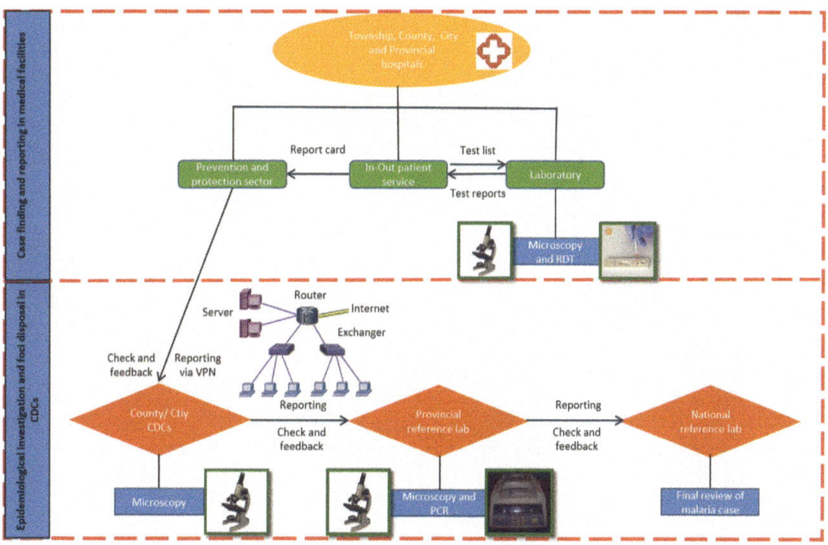

Fig. 4 Malaria surveillance and response network systems in Jiangsu Province.

Note: Jiangsu provincial malaria surveillance and response network systems covers case finding and reporting in all levels of medical facilities and epidemiological investigation and foci disposals in CDCs. When a fever patient went to hospital, the suspected case will be received blood test or/and RDT. Once confirmed, the relevant information of malaria case will be reported through CISDCP and China's 1-3-7 approach would be initiated and take rapid response.

4.1 Case reporting within 1 day

In Jiangsu Province, since the initialization of the 1-3-7 surveillance and response approach in 2012, a total number of 2423 malaria cases were detected and reported from 2012 to 2020. All 2423 cases were reported within 1 day (24h) through CISDCP reporting system (Table 1).

These 2423 malaria cases include 1884 *falciparum* malaria cases, 84 *vivax* malaria cases, 347 *ovale* malaria cases, 87 *malariae* malaria cases and 21 mixed infection cases. They were distributed in 90 counties of 13 cities in Jiangsu Province. A large number of the reported cases were from Nantong city (366 cases, accounting for 15.11%), Lianyungang city (287 cases, accounting for 11.84%), Taizhou city (282 cases, accounting for 11.64%), Yangzhou city (277 cases, accounting for 11.43%), Huai'an city (267 cases, accounting for 11.02%), and Nanjing city (178 cases, accounting for 7.35%) (Fig. 5).

Table 1 Number of cases with different species distributed by year from 2012 to 2020.

Year	*P. faciparum*	*P. vivax*	*P. ovale*	*P. malariae*	Mixed infection	Total
2012	171[a]	4	19	2	2	198
2013	286	8	30	9	8	341
2014	292	4	46	10	3	355
2015	299	13	71	18	4	405
2016	237	11	51	8	1	308
2017	163	21	43	11	1	239
2018	171	14	42	15	1	243
2019	206	4	22	12	0	244
2020	59	5	23	2	1	90
Total	1884	84	347	87	21	2423

[a]*Note:* Four cases were clinically diagnosed as *P. falciparum* malaria among them.

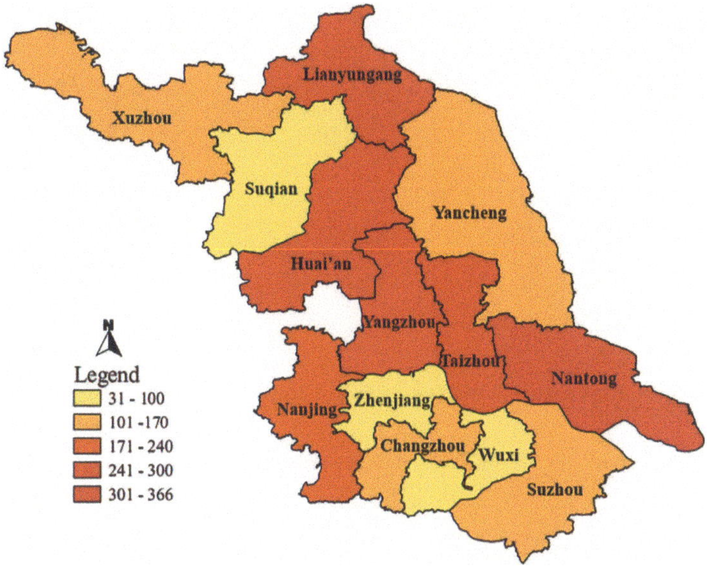

Fig. 5 Regional distribution of malaria cases in Jiangsu Province during 2012–2020.

Moreover, all the 2423 cases were totally reported by medical facilities (1732, 71.48%), CDCs (651, 26.87%) and entry-exit inspection and quarantine (China Customs at present) (40, 1.65%).

4.2 Case confirmation and classification within 3 days

A cell phone-based short message service alert system has been used to immediately inform local CDC staff when a case is found, ensuring timely follow-up. Moreover, all the 2423 cases reported through the web-based real time reporting system were tested in the laboratories. Of which, 2419 cases (98.42%) were finally lab-confirmed, and 4 cases (1.58%) were clinically diagnosed, which were reported in 2012 in the early phase of implementing the 1-3-7 approach. Of the 2419 lab-confirmed cases, 1880 were *P. falciparum* (77.72%), 84 were *P. vivax* (3.47%), 347 were *P. ovale* (14.34%), 87 were *P. malariae* (3.60%) and 21 were mixed infections (0.87%) (Fig. 6). It is seen that more than 98% of malaria cases received individual epidemiological investigations by local CDC staff at the county level within 3 days (Table 2).

According to the implementation of the 1-3-7 surveillance and response approach from 2012 to 2020, of the totally reported 2423 malaria cases in Jiangsu Province, 2359 were males and 64 were females, with a

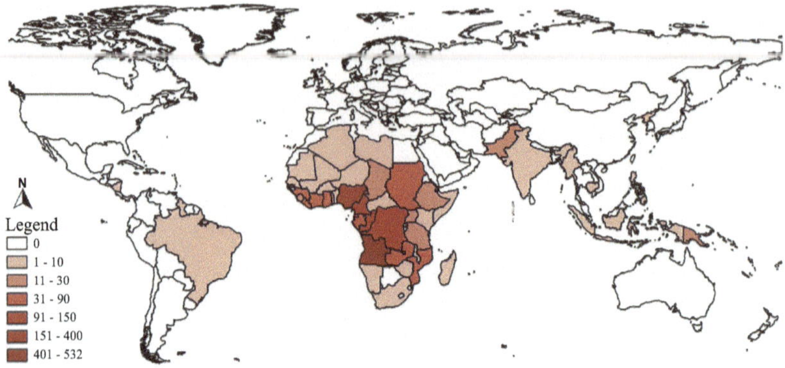

Fig. 6 Origins distribution of malaria cases in Jiangsu Province during 2012–2020.

male-female ratio of 36.86:1; the age was ranged between 2 and 71 years old, with an average age of 42.24; the main occupation of the patients was migrant workers, among which farmers, mobile workers and labourers accounted for 94.3% of the total cases.

Among the 2423 malaria cases in the province from 2012 to 2020, all malaria cases in Jiangsu Province were imported abroad. Also, there were four transfusion-transmitted malaria cases through receiving mobile labourers' blood donation (Zhang et al., 2020). An induced case refers to a case for which the origin can be traced to blood transfusion or other form of parenteral inoculation of the parasite but not to transmission by a natural mosquito-borne inoculation (WHO, 2017). In Jiangsu Province, all the other 2419 malaria cases from 52 countries and regions, among which 2360 cases were infected in Africa (97.56%), 55 cases were infected in Southeast Asia (2.27%), and four cases were infected in South America (0.17%) (Fig. 6).

4.3 Focus investigation and action within 7 days

In accordance with China Technical Scheme of Malaria Elimination, Jiangsu Province issued provincial malaria elimination surveillance programme and Jiangsu annual work programme of malaria elimination. Jiangsu Province implemented different actions in which triggered according to the results of the investigation and should be completed within 7 days. The focus/foci classification refers to the periods between case investigation and foci disposal. The focus/foci can be divided into the following three types: (1) Focus where transmission has occurred with existed transmission: natural villages (resident groups) with imported secondary transmission cases.

Table 2 Indicators of the 1-3-7 approach in Jiangsu Province, 2012–2020.

	Case detection and notification			Case investigation		Focus investigation and action	
Year	**Number of imported malaria cases**	**Number of cases reported within 1 day**	**Proportion of cases reported within 1 day**	**Number of cases investigated within 3 days**	**Proportion of cases investigated within 3 days**	**Number of foci investigations and action taken within 7 days**	**Proportion of foci investigations and action taken within 7 days**
2012	198	198	100.00%	193	98.97%	191	96.46%
2013	341	341	100.00%	341	100.00%	341	100.00%
2014	355	355	100.00%	355	100.00%	355	100.00%
2015	405	405	100.00%	405	100.00%	405	100.00%
2016	308	308	100.00%	308	100.00%	308	100.00%
2017	239	239	100.00%	231	97.91%	223	93.31%
2018	243	243	100.00%	242	99.59%	240	98.77%
2019	244	244	100.00%	244	100.00%	238	97.54%
2020	90	90	100.00%	90	100.00%	81	90.00%
合计	2423	2423	100.00%	2409	99.42%	2382	98.31%

(2) Focus/foci with possible transmission: natural villages (resident groups) with imported cases and transmission conditions, and natural villages (resident groups) where imported *P. vivax* were found from May to October in Jiangsu Province. (3) Focus/foci without transmission possibility: natural villages (resident groups) without malaria vectors or with malaria vectors but not in the malaria-transmitted seasons when imported malaria cases occurred, natural villages (resident groups) where all imported *P. falciparum*, *P. ovale* and *P. malariae* as well as imported *P. vivax* cases in non-epidemic seasons located. From 2012 to 2020, the number of foci investigations and action taken within 7 days were 2382 and the proportion of foci investigations and action taken within 7 days was 98.31%, where effectively blocked the spread of malaria (Table 2).

For example, from 2012 to 2020, a total of 84 cases of *P. vivax* were reported in Jiangsu Province. Among them, 50 cases of *P. vivax* were reported during from May to October each year. And, they were distributed in 13 prefectures in Jiangsu, including seven cases in Nanjing city, six cases in Xuzhou city, six cases in Suzhou city, five cases in Lianyungang city, four cases in Changzhou city, four cases in Nantong city, three cases in Wuxi city, three cases in Yangzhou city, three cases in Taizhou city, three case in Huai'an city, three case in Zhenjiang city, two cases in Yancheng city, and one case in Suqian city. All of them were investigated and disposed as focus/foci with potential for transmission within 7 days. The measures of focus/foci disposal composed of *plasmodium* tests for fever patients, infection sources cleared in local residents, transmission vector control and population health education. The remaining 2339 cases were all focus/foci with no potential for transmission during 2012 to 2020.

5. Challenges for implementing malaria 1-3-7 approach in Jiangsu Province

5.1 The sensitivity of the malaria surveillance system needs to be improved

During malaria elimination, the surveillance system is capable to detect both symptomatic and asymptomatic cases in the community and timely treat each malaria case in order to block any potential transmission. When countries are scaling up malaria interventions towards elimination, it demands on malaria diagnostics from diagnosing ill patients to detecting parasites in all carriers including asymptomatic infections and infections with low parasite densities (Harris et al., 2010). Detection of all infected persons, including asymptomatic carriers with low and sub-microscopic parasite densities is critical to the elimination of malaria, as these carriers harbour a parasite reservoir in the population which can still potently be transmitted to mosquitoes and contribute to human transmission (Tadesse et al., 2018). In Jiangsu Province, the main diagnostic tool in health facilities at the county and township levels is light microscopy. However, the sensitivity of microscopy, the traditional method used for diagnosing *Plasmodium* infections, is frequently insufficient for detecting asymptomatic infections due to the low density of parasitaemia (Golassa et al., 2015; Tadesse et al., 2015; Zaw et al., 2017). Moreover, the challenges associated with the microscopy (e.g., availability of skilled microscopists, maintenance of technical equipment, systematic quality control) are also noticed in other malaria elimination settings (Turki et al., 2015). Jiangsu Province has adopted multiplex PCR, real-time PCR and loop-mediated isothermal amplification (LAMP) to detect and diagnose *Plasmodium* infections with sub-microscopic parasite densities, while these technologies are not widely used in primary healthcare facilities (Xu et al., 2018). Therefore, more sensitive, low-cost, and easy-operation diagnostic techniques are needed to improve the sensitivity of the malaria surveillance system.

5.2 Innovative strategies in the management of mobile and migrant populations need to be implemented

As countries move towards malaria elimination, the biggest threat to the elimination efforts is the risk of resurgence due to imported malaria and the continuing receptivity in parts of the country due to the persistence of malaria vectors (Bruce-Chwatt, 1968; Dharmawardena et al., 2015; Sturrock et al., 2015). In China, imported malaria cases are mainly migrant workers coming back from SSA (Li et al., 2016). Innovative strategies, such as active surveillance activities (screening the peers of index cases) aimed at at-risk populations have been considered to be promising for early malaria case detection, particularly in counties with high numbers of imported malaria cases (Lu et al., 2016). The success of this strategy has been demonstrated in 2013 in four Chinese provinces, where the screening of 4358 peers from 167 index cases led to the detection of an additional 737 imported malaria cases (Feng et al., 2014; Mukadi et al., 2016). The proper management of imported malaria cases and mobile and migrant populations is critical to prevent malaria outbreaks and re-establishment. Therefore, mobile and migrant populations need to be systematically managed and fully incorporated in any strategies and policies to effectively progress towards elimination and prevention of re-establishment of malaria.

5.3 The delayed presentation of malaria patients to healthcare needs to be intervened

For returning international travellers with malaria, promptly seeking healthcare is extremely important for promoting early diagnosis and treatment, reducing morbidity and mortality and preventing further transmission (Liu et al., 2017; Lu et al., 2021a,b). In Jiangsu Province, malaria imported from other countries mostly occurs in adult males returning from overseas labourers (Liu et al., 2014). Previous studies have identified that one-third of the cases with imported malaria sought healthcare more than 3 days after symptom onset, which clearly represented delayed healthcare-seeking behaviour (Lu et al., 2021a,b). Similar patterns of the delayed care healthcare-seeking were also noticed from other provinces (Wang et al., 2019a,b). Therefore, the delay in seeking of medical care among migrant workers with imported malaria should be considered and addressed by specific interventions. For example, targeted pre-travel health education programme should be provided and enhanced to increase the awareness of early healthcare seeking among the migrant workers.

5.4 The malaria surveillance and response system needs to be sustained

The strong political commitment has been essential for China's achievement in bringing 30 million malaria cases a year to zero over the course of seven decades (Feng et al., 2018). However, after reaching the zero malaria milestone, there is a risk of turning attention away from the necessary actions and investments in surveillance and infection control to prevent onward malaria transmission in China. The significant decline in malaria cases has meant that professionals engaged in malaria prevention and treatment have become deficient in their skills and practice (Feng et al., 2020). When there are no indigenous malaria cases, sustaining the capacity of the disease control institutions and maintaining the diagnostic ability of healthcare workers and CDC staff remain challenging (Cao et al., 2018). Therefore, in order to maintain well functioning of the 1-3-7 approach, strengthening the political commitment and sustaining investments in the surveillance response system are critically important.

Many malaria-receptive areas remain in China, especially during the warm summer months. Continued importation of malaria across its southern border with Myanmar, and from Chinese workers returning from overseas

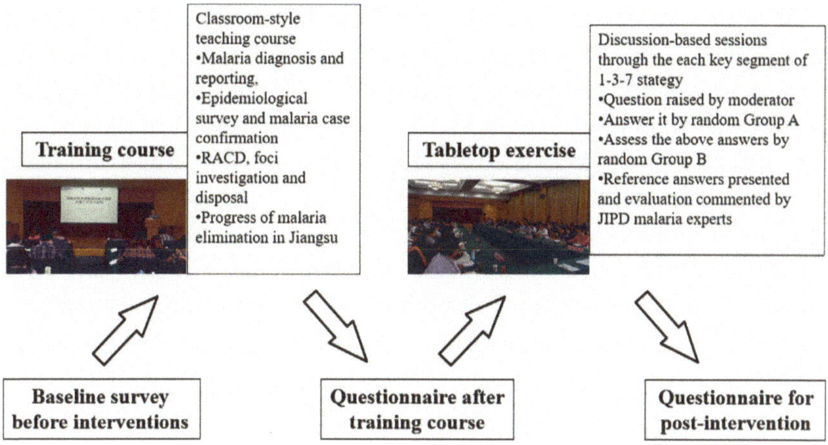

Fig. 7 Flowchart of surveys and different training modules.

is a threat to maintaining the interruption of indigenous malaria transmission in China. In 2016, in order to cope with challenge, Jiangsu Province carried out malaria training module (using classroom-style teaching) and tabletop exercises (using discussion-based sessions) with pre- and post-intervention. A total of 125 participants were selected from all 13 city CDCs and 100 county CDCs across Jiangsu Province. One to two government personnel in each county and prefecture CDC are responsible for the daily management of malaria control and other parasites. Overall, knowledge of the 1-3-7 approach for malaria elimination was 63.2% correct at baseline, 70.6% after implementing a classroom-style teaching module ($\chi^2=11.20$, $P=0.001$), and 84.6% after the tabletop exercise module ($\chi^2=48.82$, $P<0.001$). The knowledge of each component of the 1-3-7 approach improved significantly after the tabletop exercise module. More interactive and discussion based methods, such as the tabletop exercises, can increase the knowledge of basic CDC malaria personnel on China's 1-3-7 surveillance and response approach (Cao et al., 2020) (Fig. 7).

6. Lessons learned from implementing malaria 1-3-7 approach in Jiangsu Province

6.1 A well-established communicable disease reporting system is essential

China Information System for Disease Control and Prevention (CISDCP) is an internet-based real-time disease-reporting system firstly established in 2004, and has evolved to cover 55,077 national health facilities in 397 cities of all 31 provinces in the mainland of China (Wang et al., 2008). Hospital doctors are responsible for collecting and reporting the individual case information through the web-based reporting system. This Internet-based real-time disease-reporting system covering 40 notifiable diseases (*COVID-19* was included since January 2020) (Geng et al., 2021). All 40 notifiable infectious diseases were classified into three categories. A disease in category A should be reported within 2h once diagnosed. The diseases in categories B and C should be reported within 24h (Yang et al., 2017). The CISDCP begins at the township level and guarantees, to a large degree, the reporting of malaria cases within 1 day. Moreover, the well-established web-based reporting network, for example, the cell phone-based SMS alert system that promptly informs the local CDC at the county level, is extremely important in completing case investigation and taking appropriate public health responses in regulated time targets.

6.2 Strengthening of surveillance for malaria case detection by optimizing the malaria blood testing network

Jiangsu Province has established a provincial, municipal, city, county and township-level malaria blood test network, in which clinically diagnosed malaria patients, patients with suspected malaria and a fever of unknown origin ("three fevers") will all receive a malaria blood test. In Jiangsu Province, from 2011 to 2020, 3,637,562 patients with fevers received blood tests of *plasmodium*.

Moreover, in order to encourage early malaria case detection and reporting, rewards mechanism for case reporting and case verification in elimination phase was established. For example, Renminbi 50 Yuan (equivalent to USD $7.85) will be rewarded for health staff who reported one infected individual through the direct network report system, and an additional Renminbi RMB 100 Yuan (equivalent to USD $15.70) will be rewarded for the collection of blood smears, dried blood spots and anti-coagulated blood samples, completion of epidemiological investigations, and reporting all necessary information into the reporting system on time.

6.3 Strengthening malaria diagnostic capacity at primary health facilitates

At the beginning of NMEAP implementation in Jiangsu Province, although provincial surveillance and response has been well established, an insufficient capacity for malaria diagnosis was observed, especially the preparing and reading the blood smears at the township and village levels where is still a challenge to achieve and maintain malaria-free status. Therefore, regular training and supervision of microscopy skills should be provided to staff especially at the township level (Ding et al., 2018). Considering RDT which may likely to be promoted and applied in primary health facilities, Jiangsu began to pilot the application of RDT technology in city, county and township medical institutions since 2012. JIPD is responsible for purchasing RDTs and offering to local medical facilities for free in Jiangsu Province. In order to increase the diagnostic capacity in locally medical facilities, a total number of 342,400 RDTs were purchased by JIPD from 2012 to 2017. All the RDTs are distributed to local medical facilities in the jurisdiction by municipal and county CDCs. In counties and towns where a large number of people working abroad, the supply of RDTs at the grassroots level are particularity guaranteed. Moreover, an empirical evidence for RDT's Standard Operation Procedures (SOP) posters was developed in 2018 to guide the use of RDT at primary health facilities. The comprehensive package of RDT implementation in Jiangsu Province has been promising in scale up RDT use and improve access to malaria diagnosis. This implementation research provided experiences for malaria elimination settings and areas where malaria transmission is low (Liang et al., 2020).

6.4 Establishment of quality control system for malaria diagnosis

The Jiangsu Provincial Malaria Reference Laboratory affiliated to JIPD was established in 2012 and was responsible for malaria case diagnosis, confirmation and feedback. The main responsibility of the Provincial malaria reference laboratory is to check the blood smears and anticoagulated blood samples both by microscopy and PCR to confirm and classify plasmodium species. In Jiangsu Province, all blood smears, which tested and reported by the county CDCs will be further tested by the provincial reference laboratory. Moreover, all clinically diagnosed malaria patients, patients with suspected malaria, and patients with a fever of unknown origin will be further tested and confirmed in the provincial reference laboratory. In additional, a sensitive pathogen surveillance network is established in Jiangsu Province by adopting other molecular diagnostic technologies, including PCR, real-time PCR, and loop-mediated isothermal amplification (LAMP) (Lu et al., 2012).

6.5 Multisectoral coordination mechanism and management of migrant population

Since the initialization of malaria elimination in China, led by Jiangsu Commission of Health, a multisectoral and coordination mechanism was developed involving all relevant sectors in programme implementation. The key sectors include the Department of Development and Reform, the Department of Finance, the Department of Public Security, the Department of Commerce, Entry-exit Inspection and Quarantine, Jiangsu Radio and Television Bureau, the Department of Education, and the Department of Science & Technology in Jiangsu Province. The multi-sectoral and coordination mechanism is expected to jointly implement, coordinate, support, and evaluate implementation of malaria elimination programmes. In 2010, Jiangsu Provincial Government issued the *Jiangsu Province Malaria Elimination Action Plan (2010–2020)* to guide malaria elimination activities. All departments and bureaus which involved shall need to make clear objectives and measures to malaria elimination based on the Jiangsu Provincial Malaria Weekly issued by JIPD. For example, the Provincial Department of Finance gradually increased investment in malaria control and elimination. Since 2011, Jiangsu Provincial Department of Finance has invested a total of Renminbi 35 million Yuan (equivalent to USD $0.5 million) to ensure the implementation of the malaria elimination programme. Another example is that Jiangsu Radio and Television Bureau played pivotal roles in promoting the knowledge on malaria prevention and control to the public.

Mobile and migrant populations, groups or individuals are highly vulnerable to malaria because of barriers/obstacles to access to "basic" and "quality" health-care services for both health and malaria curative and preventive services (WHO, 2015a,b). Considering the poor performance in awareness, attitudes and practices of international labourers from rural areas, professionals of malaria control and prevention are invited to provide pre-departure seminar for migrant workers who plan and apply to work abroad. For the agency hired workers, tracing and investigation of accompanies of returning migrant workers with malaria largely facilitate the early detection and diagnosis of infected individuals. Moreover, Jiangsu Entry-Exit Inspection and Quarantine Bureau (CIQ, China Customs) was actively involved in screening for entry-exit personnel for malaria. Since 2011, the entry-exit ports of Jiangsu Province have detected 36 imported malaria cases returning from the malaria highly-endemic areas in Africa and Southeast Asia.

6.6 Conducting operational research and supervision to facilitate the implementation of the 1-3-7 approach

In order to explore and solve operational challenges in implementing the 1-3-7 approach, Jiangsu Province carried out operational researches and provided scientific evidences and technical supports in eliminating malaria stage (Zhou et al., 2015). For example, since the beginning of the 1-3-7 approach, the proportion of malaria cases for which focus investigation and response occur within 7 days was only around 50% as of 2013 in China (Cao et al., 2014). The Jiangsu Province immediately carried out relevant operational researches to explore the operational challenges in the implementation 1-3-7 approach in order to enable further improvements. One of the challenges related to focus/foci investigation and response within 7 days is the lack of clear implementation guidelines for county staff on whether or not and how the focus investigation should be conducted.

In Jiangsu Province, local CDCs' malaria staffs were coordinated to supervise and inspect the activities in 1-3-7 approach. Prefectural CDCs are in charge of supervision and inspection to grass-root medical facilities in the region at least once a year. The supervision and inspection were conducted following by the administration of JIPD. Moreover, JIPD developed an annual supervision and inspection routine in type 2 counties, which were classified according to the four-catalogue classification of transmission settings based on malaria transmission risk and incidence at county level.

6.7 International exchange and cooperation

Since 2002, JIPD has successively have organized over 59 foreign-aid technical training courses and international training courses such as International Tropical Disease Control Technology Training Course and Seminar on Malaria Control for African Countries subsidized by Ministry of Commerce. More than 2000 trainees including health officials and professional technical personnel from over 70 African and Asian developing countries were trained by JIPD. During the malaria training course for these years, JIPD has organized and released diverse learning courseware, especially in strengthening the publicity and implementation of 1-3-7 approach. Cooperation with foreign aid policies, JIPD has helped developing countries train management and technical talents in the field of malaria control and prevention.

Since 2013, JIPD and University of California, San Francisco (UCSF) started to work at the secretariat of Asia Pacific Malaria Elimination

Network-Surveillance and Response Working Group (APMEN-SRWG) as the joint chairman units, and have undertaken or jointly held 6 courses of international conferences on malaria elimination in Thailand, Indonesia and China successively in which greatly promoting the malaria elimination in Asia-Pacific. Moreover, in October 2016, JIPD was appointed by WHO as the Collaborating Center (WHOCC) for Research and Training on Malaria Elimination, with main responsibilities of implementing the collection and Research and Development (R&D) of relevant malaria-eliminating strategies and technologies and conducting technical training and scientific researches related to malaria elimination, so as to provide technical support for global malaria eradication.

7. Conclusions

Jiangsu Province has established an efficient and sensitive system for case-based malaria surveillance and response to achieve malaria elimination and manage imported malaria cases returning from abroad. Maintaining knowledge of malaria among high risk groups, ensuring proper health-seeking behaviours of malaria patients, guaranteeing timely and accurate malaria diagnosis, and ensuring well implementation of real-time case reporting, timely case confirmation and rapid focus/foci disposal will be critical for Jiangsu Province and China to maintain malaria free.

Acknowledgements

This study was supported by Bill & Melinda Gates Foundation (INV-018913), the National Natural Science Foundation of China (71904165), the Jiangsu Provincial Health Commission (H2018102, and X201828), and the Jiangsu Provincial Project of Invigorating Health Care through Science, Technology, and Education.

References

Bruce-Chwatt, L.J., 1968. Movements of populations in relation to communicable disease in Africa. East Afr. Med. J. 45 (3), 266–275.

Cao, J., Sturrock, H.J., Cotter, C., Zhou, S., Zhou, H., Liu, Y., et al., 2014. Communicating and monitoring surveillance and response activities for malaria elimination: China's "1-3-7" strategy. PLoS Med. 11, e1001642.

Cao, Y.Y., Zhou, H.Y., Zhu, G.D., Wang, W.M., Jin, J.J., et al., 2018. Challenges for maintaining achievements of malaria elimination in Jiangsu Province, China [in Chinese]. Zhongguo Xue Xi Chong Bing Fang Zhi Za Zhi 30 (4), 460–464.

Cao, Y., Cotter, C., Wang, W., Liu, Y., Zhou, H., Zhu, G., et al., 2020. Malaria elimination in China: improving county-level malaria personnel knowledge of the 1-3-7 strategy through tabletop exercises. Am. J. Trop. Med. Hyg. 102 (4), 804–810.

Cohen, J.M., Smith, D.L., Cotter, C., Yamey, A.W.G., Sabot, O.J., Moonen, B., 2012. Malaria resurgence: a systematic review and assessment of its causes. Malar. J. 11, 122.

Cotter, C., Prayuth, S., Herdiana, H., Cao, Y.Y., Liu, Y.B., Luo, A., et al., 2017. Piloting a programme tool to evaluate malaria case investigation and reactive case detection activities: results from 3 settings in the Asia Pacific. Malar. J. 16, 347.

Dharmawardena, P., Premaratne, R.G., Gunasekera, W.M., Hewawitarane, M., Mendis, K., Fernando, D., 2015. Characterization of imported malaria, the largest threat to sustained malaria elimination from Sri Lanka. Malar. J. 14, 177.

Ding, G., Zhu, G., Cao, C., Miao, P., Cao, Y., Wang, W., et al., 2018. The challenge of maintaining microscopist capacity at basic levels for malaria elimination in Jiangsu Province, China. BMC Public Health 18 (1), 489.

Feng, X.Y., Xia, Z.G., Vong, S., Yang, W.Z., Zhou, S.S., 2014. Surveillance and response to drive the national malaria elimination program. Adv. Parasitol. 86, 81–108.

Feng, J., Xiao, H., Xia, Z., Zhang, L., Xiao, N., 2015. Analysis of malaria epidemiological characteristics in the People's Republic of China, 2004–2013. Am. J. Trop. Med. Hyg. 93 (2), 293–299.

Feng, J., Zhang, L., Huang, F., Yin, J.H., Tu, H., Xia, Z.G., et al., 2018. Ready for malaria elimination: zero indigenous case reported in the People's Republic of China'. Malar. J. 17, 315.

Feng, X., Levens, J., Zhou, X.N., 2020. Protecting the gains of malaria elimination in China. Infect. Dis. Poverty 9 (1), 43.

Geng, M.J., Zhang, H.Y., Yu, L.J., Lv, C.L., Wang, T., Che, T.L., et al., 2021. Changes in notifiable infectious disease incidence in China during the COVID-19 pandemic. Nat. Commun. 12, 6923.

Golassa, L., Baliraine, F.N., Enweji, N., Erko, B., Swedberg, G., Aseffa, A., 2015. Microscopic and molecular evidence of the presence of asymptomatic *Plasmodium falciparum* and *Plasmodium vivax* infections in an area with low, seasonal and unstable malaria transmission in Ethiopia. BMC Infect. Dis. 15, 310.

Harris, I., Sharrock, W.W., Bain, L.M., Gray, K.A., Bobogare, A., Boaz, L., et al., 2010. A large proportion of asymptomatic Plasmodium infections with low and sub-microscopic parasite densities in the low transmission setting of Temotu Province, Solomon Islands: challenges for malaria diagnostics in an elimination setting. Malar. J. 9, 254.

Hsiang, M.S., Hwang, J., Tao, A.R., Liu, Y.B., Bennett, A., Shanks, G.D., et al., 2013. Mass drug administration for the control and elimination of *Plasmodium vivax* malaria: an ecological study from Jiangsu province, China. Malar. J. 12 (1), 383.

Jiangsu Commission of Health, 2016. Jiangsu Health Yearbook.

Jiangsu Provincial People's Government, 2010. Jiangsu Malaria Elimination Action Plan (2010–2020). http://www.jiangsu.gov.cn/art/2010/9/13/art_46144_2544815.html. Accessed in 15 Dec 2021.

Jiangsu Provincial People's Government, 2021. http://en.jiangsu.gov.cn/col/col54121/index.html. Accessed in 15 Dec 2021.

Li, Z., Zhang, Q., Zheng, C., Zhou, S., Sun, J., Zhang, Z., et al., 2016. Epidemiologic features of overseas imported malaria in the People's Republic of China. Malar. J. 15, 141.

Liang, D., Jin, J.J., Wang, W.M., Cao, Y.Y., Zhu, G.D., Zhou, H.Y., et al., 2020. Evaluating the implementation of rapid diagnostic tests in a malaria elimination setting. Infectious Diseases of Poverty 9, 84.

Liu, Y.B., Hsiang, M.S., Zhou, H.Y., Wang, W.M., Cao, Y.Y., Gosling, R.D., et al., 2014. Malaria in overseas labourers returning to China: an analysis of imported malaria in Jiangsu Province, 2001–2011. Malar. J. 13, 29.

Liu, Y., Sturrock, H., Yang, H., Gosling, R.D., Cao, J., 2017. The challenge of imported malaria to eliminating countries. Lancet Infect. Dis. 17 (2), 141.

Lu, F., Gao, Q., Zhou, H., Cao, J., Wang, W., Lim, C.S., et al., 2012. Molecular test for vivax malaria with loop-mediated isothermal amplification method in central China. Parasitol. Res. 110 (6), 2439–2444.

Lu, G., Zhou, S., Horstick, O., Wang, X., Liu, Y., Müller, O., 2014. Malaria outbreaks in China (1990–2013): a systematic review. Malar. J. 13, 269.

Lu, G., Liu, Y., Beiersmann, C., Feng, Y., Cao, J., Muller, O., 2016. Challenges in and lessons learned during the implementation of the 1-3-7 malaria surveillance and response strategy in China: a qualitative study. Infect. Dis. Poverty 5 (1), 94.

Lu, G., Cao, Y., Chai, L., Li, Y., Li, S., Heuschen, A.K., et al., 2021a. Barriers to seeking health care among returning travellers with malaria: a systematic review. Trop. Med. Int. Health.

Lu, G., Cao, Y., Chen, Q., Zhu, G., Müller, O., Cao, J., 2021b. Care-seeking delay of imported malaria to China: implications for improving post-travel healthcare for migrant workers. J. Travel Med.

Ma, J.Q., Wang, L.P., Qi, X.P., Shi, X.M., Yang, G.H., 2006. The conceptual model of the automatic early-warning system of infectious diseases. Ji Bing Jian Ce 21 (12), 679–681.

Ma, J.Q., Wang, L.P., Qi, X.P., Shi, X.M., Yang, G.H., 2007. Conceptual model for automatic early warning information system of infectious diseases based on internet reporting surveillance system. Biomed. Environ. Sci. 20 (3), 208–211.

Moonen, B., Cohen, J.M., Snow, R.W., Slutsker, L., Drakeley, C., Smith, D.L., et al., 2010. Operational strategies to achieve and maintain malaria elimination. Lancet 376 (8752), 1592–1603.

Mukadi, P., Lejon, V., Barbé, B., Gillet, P., Nyembo, C., Lukuka, A., et al., 2016. Performance of microscopy for the diagnosis of malaria and human African trypanosomiasis by diagnostic laboratories in the Democratic Republic of the Congo: results of a nation-wide external quality assessment. PLoS One 11, e0146450.

National Health Commission of the People's Republic of China, 2010. National Malaria Elimination Action Plan (2010–2020). http://www.nhc.gov.cn/zwgk/wtwj/201304/15a4cc7a40b0452191fe409590ca99d8.shtml. Accessed in 15 Dec 2021.

Shang, L.Y., Gao, Q., Liu, X., Shen, Y.Z., Huang, G.Q., 2006. Evaluation oil the effect of cooperative malaria control in 5 provinces of central China in 30 years. Zhongguo Bing Yuan Sheng Wu Xue Za Zhi 1 (1), 51–54.

Sturrock, H.J.W., Roberts, K.W., Wegbreit, J., Ohrt, C., Gosling, R.D., 2015. Tackling imported malaria: an elimination endgame. Am. J. Trop. Med. Hyg. 93 (1), 139–144.

Tadesse, F.G., Pett, H., Baidjoe, A., Lanke, K., Grignard, L., Sutherland, C., et al., 2015. Submicroscopic carriage of *Plasmodium falciparum* and *Plasmodium vivax* in a low endemic area in Ethiopia where no parasitaemia was detected by microscopy or rapid diagnostic test. Malar. J. 14, 303.

Tadesse, F.G., Slater, H.C., Chali, W., Teelen, K., Lanke, K., Belachew, M., et al., 2018. The relative contribution of symptomatic and asymptomatic *Plasmodium vivax* and *Plasmodium falciparum* infections to the infectious reservoir in a low-endemic setting in Ethiopia. Clin. Infect. Dis. 66, 1883–1891.

Turki, H., Raeisi, A., Malekzadeh, K., Ghanbarnejad, A., Zoghi, S., Yeryan, M., et al., 2015. Efficiency of nested-PCR in detecting asymptomatic cases toward malaria elimination program in an endemic area of Iran. Iran. J. Parasitol. 10, 39–45.

Wang, L., Wang, Y., Jin, S., Wu, Z., Chin, D.P., Koplan, J.P., et al., 2008. Emergence and control of infectious diseases in China. Lancet 372, 1598–1605.

Wang, T., Zhou, S.S., Feng, J., Yang, M.M., Chen, J., Yan, C.F., Zhang, Y., et al., 2019a. Monitoring and evaluation of intervals from onset of fever to diagnosis before "1-3-7" approach in malaria elimination: a retrospective study in Shanxi Province, China from 2013 to 2018. Malar. J. 18, 235.

Wang, W.M., Zhou, H.Y., Cao, Y.Y., Gu, Y.P., Xu, S., Zhu, G.D., et al., 2019b. Epidemiological analysis of malaria prevalence in Jiangsu Province in 2017. Zhongguo Xue Xi Chong Bing Fang Zhi Za Zhi 31 (2), 178–181.

Wang, W.M., Cao, Y.Y., Yang, M.M., Gu, Y.P., Xu, S., Zhou, H.Y., et al., 2020. Epidemic situation of malaria in Jiangsu Province in 2019 [in Chinese]. Zhongguo Xue Xi Chong Bing Fang Zhi Za Zhi 33, 411–413.

WHO, 2006. Communicable Disease Surveillance and Response Systems: Guide to Monitoring and Evaluating. https://apps.who.int/iris/handle/10665/69331?show=full.
WHO, 2015a. Mobile and Migrant Populations and Malaria Information Systems.
WHO, 2015b. Global Technical Strategy for Malaria 2016–2030.
WHO, 2017. A Framework for Malaria Elimination.
WHO, 2021. 'From 30 Million Cases to Zero China is Certified Malaria-Free by WHO. https://www.who.int/news/item/30-06-2021-from-30-million-cases-to-zero-china-is-certified-malaria-free-by-who.
Xu, S., Gu, Y.P., Cao, Y.Y., Wang, W.M., Tang, J.X., et al., 2018. Results analysis of Jiangsu provincial malaria diagnostic reference laboratory in 2017. Zhongguo Xue Xi Chong Bing Fang Zhi Za Zhi 30 (6), 630–634.
Yang, S., Wu, J., Ding, C., Cui, Y., Zhou, Y., Li, Y., et al., 2017. Epidemiological features of and changes in incidence of infectious diseases in China in the first decade after the SARS outbreak: an observational trend study. Lancet Infect. Dis. 17, 716–725.
Zaw, M.T., Thant, M., Hlaing, T.M., Aung, N.Z., Thu, M., Phumchuea, K., et al., 2017. Asymptomatic and sub-microscopic malaria infection in Kayah State, eastern Myanmar. Malar. J. 16, 138.
Zhang, L., Wilson, D.P., 2012. Trends in notifiable infectious diseases in China: implications for surveillance and population health policy. PLoS One 7, e31076.
Zhang, L., Feng, J., Xia, Z.G., 2014. Malaria situation in the People's Republic of China in 2013 [in Chinese]. Zhongguo Ji Sheng Chong Xue Yu Ji Sheng Chong Bing Za Zhi 32 (6), 407–413.
Zhang, H., Wang, L., Lai, S., Li, Z., Sun, Q., Zhang, P., 2017. Surveillance and early warning systems of infectious disease in China: from 2012 to 2014. Int. J. Health Plann. Manage. 32, 329–338.
Zhang, M.H., Xu, S., Gu, Y.P., Liu, Y.B., Lin, H., Xie, C.Y., et al., 2020. Classification of induced malaria case in an elimination setting: investigation of transfusion-transmitted malaria cases. Malar. J. 19 (1), 136.
Zheng, Q., Vanderslott, S., Jiang, B., Xu, L.L., Liu, C.S., Huo, L.L., et al., 2013. Research gaps for three main tropical diseases in the People's Republic of China. Infect. Dis. Poverty 2, 15.
Zhou, H.Y., Cao, J., Wang, W.M., Li, J.L., Gu, Y.P., Zhu, G.D., 2009a. Epidemic and control of malaria in Jiangsu Province. Zhongguo Xue Xi Chong Bing Fang Zhi Za Zhi 21 (6), 503–506.
Zhou, S.S., Wang, Y., Fang, W., Tang, L.H., 2009b. Malaria situation in the People's Republic of China in 2008. Zhongguo Ji Sheng Chong Xue Yu Ji Sheng Chong Bing Za Zhi 27 (457), 55–56.
Zhou, H.Y., Wang, W.M., Liu, Y.B., Cao, J., Gao, Q., 2012. Epidemiological analysis of malaria prevalence in Jiangsu Province in 2010. Zhongguo Xue Xi Chong Bing Fang Zhi Za Zhi 24 (3), 322–325.
Zhou, H.Y., Cao, J., Wang, W.M., Liu, Y.B., Cao, Y.Y., Gao, Q., 2013. Epidemiological analysis of malaria prevalence in Jiangsu Province in 2011. Zhongguo Xue Xi Chong Bing Fang Zhi Za Zhi 25 (1), 31–35.
Zhou, S.S., Zhang, S.S., Zhang, L., Rietveld, A.E., Ramsay, A.R., Zachariah, R., et al., 2015. China's 1-3-7 surveillance and response strategy for malaria elimination: is case reporting, investigation and foci response happening according to plan? Infect. Dis. Poverty 4, 55.
Zhou, S., Li, Z., Cotter, C., Zheng, C., Zhang, Q., Li, H., et al., 2016. Trends of imported malaria in China 2010-2014: analysis of surveillance data. Malar. J. 15, 39.
Zhu, G., Zhou, H., Li, J., Tang, J., Bai, L., Wang, W., et al., 2014. The colonization of pyrethroid resistant strain from wild Anopheles sinensis, the major Asian malaria vector. Parasit. Vectors 7, 582.

CHAPTER TWO

Historical review of malaria control and elimination in the border areas of China: A case study of Yunnan Province

Hui Liu, Yao-Wu Zhou, Yan Deng, Zu-Rui Lin, Cang-Lin Zhang, Qi-Yan Chen, Chun Wei, Kai-Xia Duan, Hong-Ning Zhou*, and Jian-wei Xu

Yunnan Institute of Parasitic Diseases, Yunnan Provincial Centre of Malaria Research, Yunnan Provincial Key Laboratory of Vector-borne Diseases Control and Research, Yunnan Institute of Parasitic Diseases Innovative Team of Key Techniques for Vector Borne Disease Control and Prevention, Training Base of International Scientific Exchange and Education in Tropical Diseases for South and Southeast Asia, Puer, Yunnan, PR China

*Corresponding author: e-mail address: zhouhn66@163.com

Contents

1. Introduction 34
2. Background 35
3. Malaria control from hyperendemicity to elimination 36
   3.1 Malaria situation and control prior to the founding of People's Republic of China 36
   3.2 Health system establishment and widespread interventions, 1950–65 39
   3.3 Malaria resurgence and epidemic control, 1966–77 41
   3.4 Consolidating and scaling up achievement, 1978–2002 43
   3.5 Malaria from control to pre-elimination, 2003–2013 48
   3.6 Malaria elimination 2014–16 50
   3.7 Preventing reintroduction and certificating malaria free 2017–June 2021 50
4. Experiences 51
   4.1 High political commitment 52
   4.2 Updated strategy in each phase of the malaria program 52
   4.3 Innovative malaria treatment schemes in the malaria program 53
   4.4 Improved information system supports surveillance and response to malaria 54
   4.5 Engagement of the broader communities 55
   4.6 Cross-border collaboration and communication 55
   4.7 Interaction between control effectiveness and socioeconomic development 56
5. Lessons 58
   5.1 The sustainability of the malaria control program needs a political stability 58
   5.2 The malaria control and elimination needs multi-sector collaboration 59

Advances in Parasitology, Volume 116
ISSN 0065-308X
https://doi.org/10.1016/bs.apar.2021.12.001

5.3 The reduction of malaria burden in border areas of neighbour countries needs cross-border collaboration at the local level 59
5.4 The effective malaria control and elimination program need prompt finding and rapid responses to malaria foci 60
5.5 The sensitivity of surveillance and response system determines the program quality in the elimination stage 60
6. Challenges and recommendations 61
6.1 Challenges 61
6.2 Recommendations 63
7. Conclusions 64
Acknowledgements 65
References 65

Abstract

To understand how malaria could be eliminated in the original hyperendmic area for malaria along international borders in Yunnan Province, malaria situation and control were described on the basis of seven phases. At last the experiences and lessons of the program that reduced border malaria from hyperendmicity to malaria-free status were summarized. Malaria control and elimination area were particularly difficult in the Yunnan border. The achievement can be attributed to high political commitment, strategic and technical innovations based on the actual locality, effective collaboration and communication with neighbouring countries to carry out cross border interventions. Other border areas might perform their own pilot interventions based on their local context, including malaria burden, governing system, health service structure contextualized based on their socioeconomic development and ecology, and then a local decision could be made according to their own trial results.

1. Introduction

Malaria is an ancient *Plasmodium* spp. disease that is transmitted by anopheline mosquitoes. Malaria has been closely accompanied with human being from beginning of human history (Alonso and Tanner, 2013). In most parts of China, including Yunnan, people commonly named malaria as "Da Bai Zi." In the South of Yunnan Province, malaria was also named "Zhang Qi" in which "Zhang" represents damp and hot bad air, and "Qi" also represents air (Yao et al., 1936; Zhang, 2005). As one of major public health problems, malaria was ever seriously hindering socioeconomic development in the People's Republic of China (P. R. China), especially in Yunnan Province (Diouf et al., 2014; Tang et al., 1991). China borders 14 countries: on the east, Russia and North Korea; on the north, Mongolia; on the west, Tajikistan, Kyrgyzstan, Kazakhstan, Pakistan, and Afghanistan; and on the south, India, Nepal, Bhutan, Myanmar, Laos, and Vietnam. Many these countries are malaria endemic, but Myanmar, Laos, and Vietnam have significant malaria impact on China among the 14 countries (Xu et al., 2021a,b. China has 34 provincial administrative regions (ethnic autonomous region or province-level municipality or special administrative region). Only Yunnan in the southwestern China is facing the problem of border malaria seriously. Yunnan Province borders with Myanmar, Laos and Vietnam. Yunnan is also a province of "ethnic minority, border, mountainous and poverty-stricken" (Yang and Zhou, 2015). The complex topography and natural environment, combined with multiple climatic zones lead to the complexity of malaria vectors, and benefit the growth and reproduction of anopheline mosquitoes and the transmission of malaria parasites. The underdeveloped socioeconomic situation, and naturally geographical and climate factors defined as Yunnan, especially border areas, was highly endemic for malaria (Xu and Liu, 1997, 2012; Xu et al., 2015). Malaria control and elimination was truly difficult in the Yunnan border area, but vitally important for China. Border malaria is one of the most intractable problems in the path to malaria elimination worldwide (World Health Organization [WHO], 2014). Malaria in the Yunnan border area definitely impaired its elimination in China. Border malaria elimination also significantly contributed to the WHO malaria elimination certification for China (Xu et al., 2021a,b). The objective of this case study is to present a picture in malaria from hyperendemicity prior to the founding of P. R. China to malaria free status when the WHO has awarded a malaria-free certification to China on June 30, 2021.

2. Background

Yunnan is a unique province with a malaria ecology and vector system similar to those of five other countries in the Great Mekong Sub region (Cui et al., 2012). A population of 48 million people scatters in 129 counties, 16 prefectures or municipalities. Among them, 909,308 people (2020) live in 8 prefectures containing 25 border counties along the 4060km international borders. The Yunnan landform is mostly vertical and mountainous, altitudes ranging from 76.4 to 6740m. The people of 13 indigenous ethnic minorities live across the boundary. The original hyperendemicity was defined by unique malaria ecology, diversity in vector species and tremendous spatial heterogeneity in the Yunnan border area. All four of the malaria parasites, namely *P. falciparum, P. vivax, P. malariae* and *P. ovale,* were identified in the area. A total of eight species of anopheline mosquitoes were identified playing roles in malaria transmission in Yunnan Province.

They are *Anopheles minimus* (primary vector), *Anopheles sinensis, Anopheles kunmingensis, Anopheles anthropophagus, and Anopheles dirus, Anopheles jeyporiensis, Anopheles pseudowillmori, Anopheles maculatus*. In most parts of the Yunnan border area, two or more malaria vectors coexist, and the vector anopheline mosquitoes have a long time of activity, biting for more than 10 months in a year. In 1953, a total of 410 thousand malaria cases were reported in Yunnan, and 164 thousand (40%) of them were from the border areas (Yang and Zhou, 2015). There were no natural or artificial barriers along the international borders prior to the corona virus disease (COVID-19) pandemic. There are 5 national, 12 provincial and 226 unofficial border crossing sites on the boundary now. It was estimated approximately 10 million people were moving around in the border area. Many of them were non immunes from the inland areas of Yunnan and other provinces in China. The migrants include Chinese people who went neighbouring countries and then returned home, foreigners who crossed the boundary for working, trading and visiting friends and relatives in China, and a large number of internal migrants who came from the inland areas in China for similar reasons each year (Xu and Liu, 1997). Internal and cross border migrants had a high morbidity and mortality before 2003 when intensive interventions for malaria were carried out. Most parts of in the Yunnan border area are tropical or subtropical climate. The development of tropical agriculture including growing rubber, tea and tropical fruits attracted a large amount of migrant farm workers who were usually from inland non-malarious areas and then suffered malaria seriously when they stayed in the border area (Xu and Liu, 1997). The border area in China is still a developing area with poor communities, marginalized populations and weak health systems. The border areas of the three neighbouring countries present year-round malaria transmission and high density of malaria vector due to lacking of control measures. The civil unrest, unpermitted border crossers and high malaria prevalence in the border area of Myanmar increased malaria cross border transmission. Each of these factors made malaria difficult to control and challenged the feasibility of malaria elimination in the Yunnan border area (Xu and Liu, 1997, 2012; Xu et al., 2015).

3. Malaria control from hyperendemicity to elimination

3.1 Malaria situation and control prior to the founding of People's Republic of China

Prior to the founding of P. R. China, there were no systemic records of malaria due to lacking of a functional system to collect data of malaria epidemiology and control activities (Song, 2008). Data for malaria burden and interventions can only be obtained from some fragmental records in literatures. For example, a book "Beginning and ending of Yunnan–Vietnam Railway" reported about 70 thousand of deaths occurred due to malaria, hungry and violence during the construction of the Yunnan-Vietnam Railway (Xu et al., 2017). The description of literatures is that "a railway crosstie, a human life; a railway spike, a drop of human blood" (Hekou Center for Diseases Control and Prevention, 2015). A folk says "Marry out your wife first if you want to go to Simao City." This is a true portrayal of the malaria epidemic in Simao City (Puer City at present) (Liang, 1940). The meaning was that a man had better divorce his wife and let her get a new husband before he left home for Simao City. The malaria epidemic in Simao City reduced the population from 70 thousand of residents in 1919 to less than one thousand in 1949 (Liang, 1940). An investigation was conducted by Dr Hou who was born in Simao City and graduated from the Shanghai Southeast Medical University and worked in Yunnan Military Hospital in Kunming. The investigation result indicated 72.9% of malaria prevalence in 1935 (Hou, 1938). The literatures reported that imported *P. falciparum* malaria by army soldiers returning from the border area caused the epidemic in Simao City due to lacking of Public health service. At that time, diseases, like malaria, were mainly treated by the private clinics of traditional Chinese medicine and herbal medicine, and resorted assistance from the ghosts and the gods (Song, 2008). In the early stage of Simao's malaria epidemic, at least one person was ill in a family; and then at least one died in a family; by the end of the epidemic the situation became more serious, in some sites all family members and all people in a village or street died out (Liang, 1940). At last Simao became an empty city, which houses and streets became weedy and bushy (Fig. 1) (Zhou et al., 2022).

To support construction of Yunnan-Myanmar Railway against Japanese invasion, the Health Department of Kuomintang Government Carried out two cross-sectional studies in 1935 and 1939, respectively. Result of the study in Southern Yunnan reported 56.1% of splenomegaly rate and 68.2 of parasite prevalence among 289 children of less than 12 years old in 1935 (Yao et al., 1936). Result of another study in Western Yunnan showed 20.1% of splenomegaly rate and 22.5 of parasite prevalence among 1620 children of less than 14 years old in 1939 (Wu, 1941). The results of the two studies also indicated that the closer to the border, the higher malaria prevalence (Wu, 1941; Yao et al., 1936). The 25th medical team of the Health Department of Kuomintang Government established a Medical Institution at Zhefang Town, Mengshi (one of border counties in Western Yunnan)

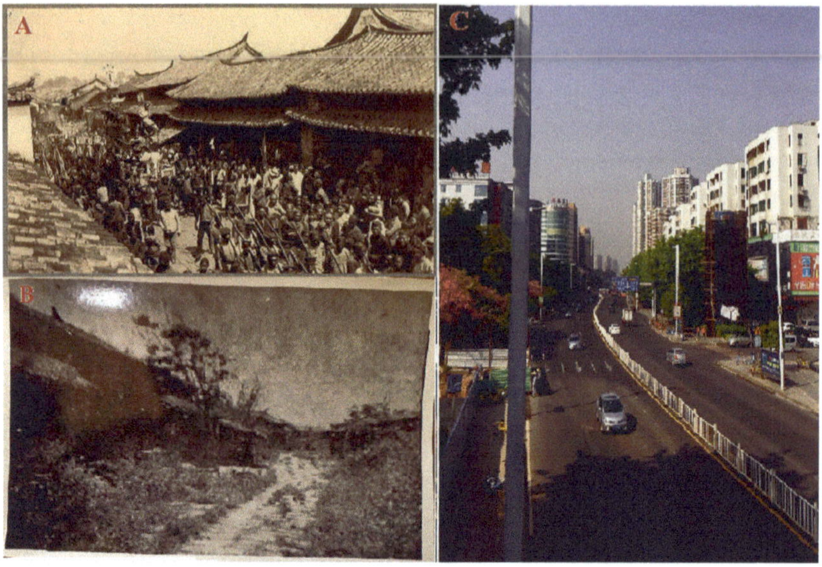

Fig. 1 The pictures of Simao streets in three eras: (A) A picture taken in 1908 to show the prosperous street prior to the epidemic of malaria; (B) A picture taken in March 1950 to show the weedy and bushy street after the malaria epidemic; (C) A picture taken in March 2021 to show today's street.

in 1938. The major mission of the Medical Institution was to fight malaria, so renamed as the Anti-malaria Team later (Dehong Center for Disease Control and Prevention, 2011). On the basis of the two investigations in the southern and western Yunnan, the Provincial Anti-malaria Committee was established to coordinate malaria control, and then the Anti-malaria Team in Mangshi was renamed as Malaria Research Institution in 1939 (Dehong Center for Disease Control and Prevention, 2011; Song, 2008). Six anti-malaria stations were meanwhile established in the other areas of Yunnan Province. One of them was stationed in Hekou on the China-Vietnam border, another one of them was in Mangshi on the China-Myanmar and four others were in the inland areas (Song, 2008). Malaria control interventions included outreach services for malaria diagnosis and treatment, distributing antimalarial drugs such as quinine and quinacrine tablets for prophylaxis, and mobilizing railway construction workers and local resident to promote housing conditions and use of bed nets, and killing mosquito larvae with 1% copper acetoarsenite powder (Yang and Zhou, 2015; Zheng, 1984). However, when Japanese Army occupied the south and west of Yunnan Province, the railway construction project was forced to stop in 1942 (Department of military history of Academy of Military Sciences, 1991), and then malaria control activities were forced to give up (Song, 2008; Wang and Yang, 2013).

3.2 Health system establishment and widespread interventions, 1950–65

The P. R. China began to fully administrated Yunnan Province on February 24, 1950. At beginning of the malaria control program, the Liberation Army helped out to carry out malaria control activities for local residents. The Central Government Administration Council released "The Work Protocol of Malaria Control in Ethnical Minority Areas" as the guidelines for malaria baseline survey and control in December 1951 (Tang and Gao, 2013). According the guidelines, the central government mobilized health professionals from the Central Anti-epidemic Team, the Liberation Army Anti-epidemic Team, the Southwestern Anti-epidemic Team and Yunnan Anti-epidemic Team, entering the Yunnan border area. The health professionals first recruited and trained local health staff. Then the trainers and trainees worked together to conduct an epidemiological baseline survey. At the same time they treated all malaria patients that they met and carried out pilot control trials (Wang and Yang, 2013). In 1953, the basleine survey was completed, and a primary health system for malaria control and prevntion was eastablished in the Yunnan border area (Yang and Zhou, 2015). The primary health system detected a total of 164,110 malaria cases, and reported the annual malaria incidence as high as 110.8 per 1000 person-years in the border area in 1953 (Wang and Yang, 2013). According to malaria epidemiological characteristics and vector ecology, "three mass measures," namely, mass drug administration for radical cure treatment in the low transmission season (December–February of next year), mass drug administration for preventive treatment with available antimalarial drugs and full indoor residual spraying with available insecticides in the high transmission season (May–December), were widespread used to reduce malaria burden. The annual malaria incidence was successfully reduced to 79.8 per 1000 person-years in 1955 (Wang and Yang, 2013; Yang and Zhou, 2015) (Fig. 2).

Starting in 1956, a 5-year malaria control program was usually formulated and conducted in Yunnan Province every 5 years. The first 5-year malaria control program was carried out during 1956–60. A pilot malaria control trial (called as malaria eradication trial at that time) was rolled out in Menghai County on the China-Myanmar border in May 1957. The pilot

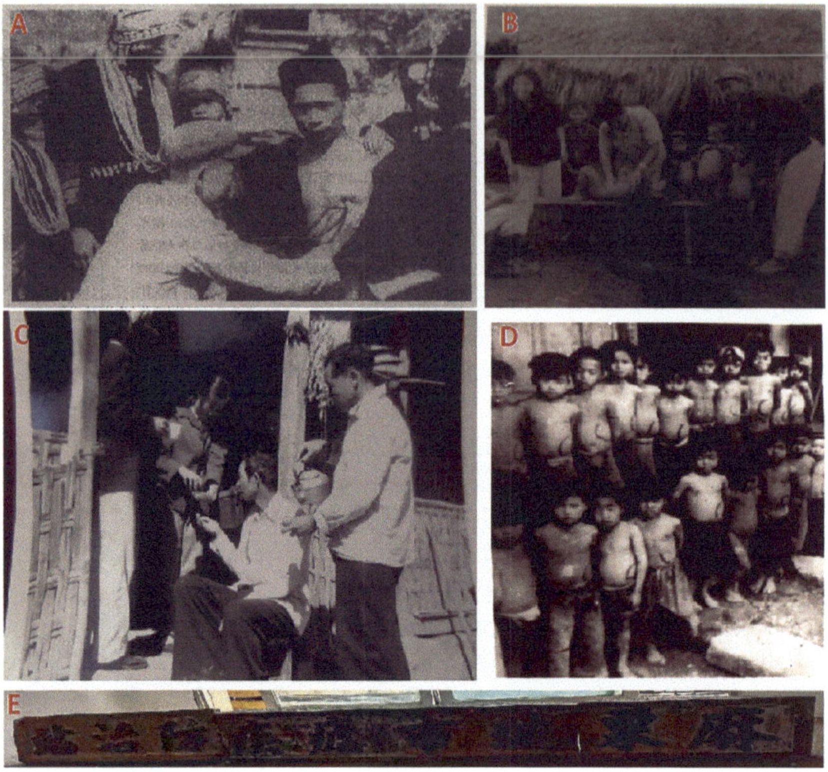

Fig. 2 Working pictures of Year 1950–65 in the Yunnan border area: (A) An army health workers was diagnosing malaria for villagers in a remote Hani ethnic minority village in Jiangcheng County on the China-Lao-Vietnam border; (B) A health workers was examining a child for splenomegaly caused by malaria in a village; (C) Health workers distribute drugs and water to people for radical cure treatment house to house; (D) A group picture taken in 1951 to show splenomegaly children with malaria infection; (E) The plaque of the Malipo City Station of Malaria Control established in 1957, renamed as the Malipo County Anti-epidemic Station later, the Malipo County Center for Disease control and Prevention at present.

trial used the "three mass measures" to successfully interrupt malaria transmission in 1962 (Wang and Yang, 2013). Based on the experiences and lessons gaining from the pilot malaria control trial, a local strategy of border malaria control was developed and then began to scale up in Yunnan Province in 1961. The strategy dynamically categorized every community into three types with high, moderate and low malaria endemic areas every year on the basis of malaria incidence in the last year. In the high endemic communities, the "three mass measures" were continuously conducted to reduce malaria burden. In the moderate and low endemic communities, the strategy was to clear parasite reservoirs first, including standardized treatment of clinical patients and parasite carriers in time, and radical cure treatment of the people who had a history of malaria attacks in the last year. Indoor residual spraying with insecticides was only carried out in the villages with the possibility of malaria transmission. Preventive treatment was only given to the people at a high risk of malaria infection, such as people who went the foot of the hill for agriculture production in the river valley area (Yang et al., 2022). Meanwhile, more new staff were recruited and intensively trained on malaria and other diseases during this phase. The capacity of health service for malaria control was further promoted. A functional health service system consisting with health facilities at three levels of county, township and village were formally established in each border county in this phase (Wang and Yang, 2013). The annual malaria incidence was successfully reduced to 4.6 per 1000 person-years in 1965 (Fig. 3).

3.3 Malaria resurgence and epidemic control, 1966–77

The number of malaria cases dropped from 9576 cases in 1965 to 7007 in 1966 in the border area. A reduction of 26.8% in the number of malaria cases detected was mostly attributable to the reduced intensity of malaria detection because of the political campaign "the Great Cultural Revolution" beginning from May 1966 (Li et al., 2017; Wang and Yang, 2013). The data could not represent actual malaria situation. From 1967, malaria gradually resurged in some malaria endemic areas (Fig. 3). More unfortunately, some border counties began to disband the County Anti-epidemic Stations or combined them into the County Hospitals in 1968. The change of the public health system led to failure to effectively implement malaria control activities. The reduced intervention intensity and the increased movement of population due to the political campaign caused a spread of malaria parasites (Wang and Yang, 2013; Xu et al., 2017). In 1971, the first two malaria epidemics took place in Yingjiang and Longling, two counties on the China-Myanmar border, respectively (Wang and Yang, 2013; Yang and Zhou, 2015). Malaria morbidity rebounded to the peak in the border area in 1973. A total of 69,473 malaria cases were reported in 1973 and the annual malaria incidence reached 23.2 per 1000 person-years. This annual malaria incidence was more than seven times of 3.2 per 1000 person-years in 1966 (Fig. 3). To control the epidemic, health staff at four levels of province, prefecture, county and township, were assigned to station in every village

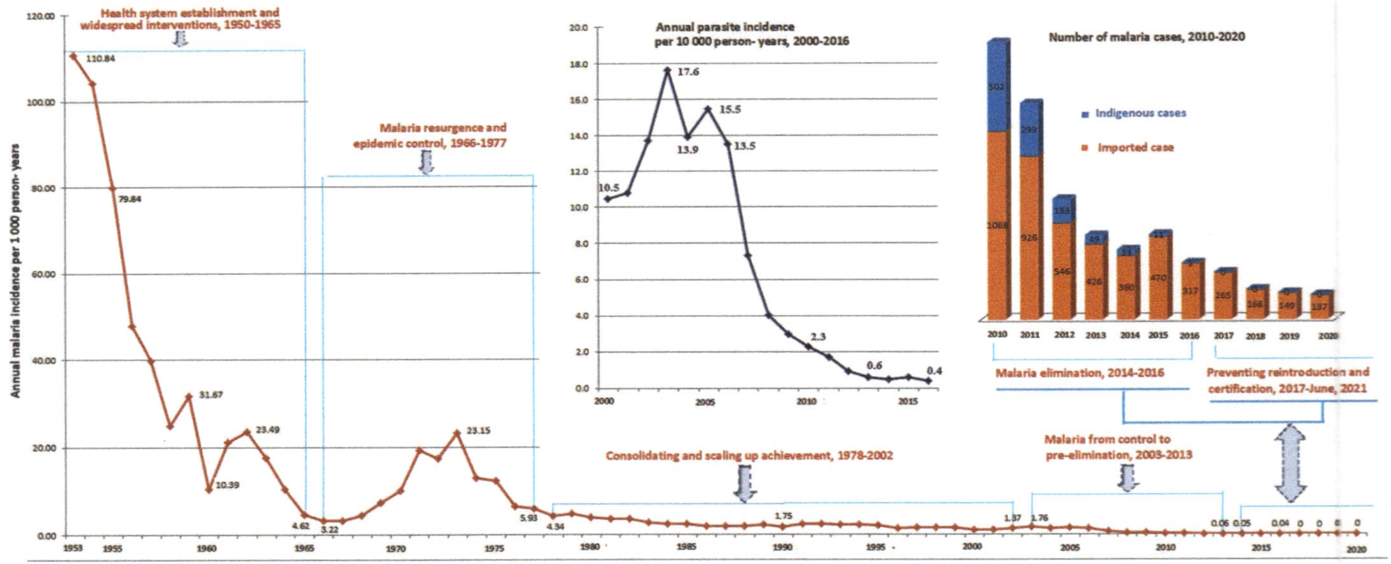

Fig. 3 The annual malaria incidence from 1953 to 2020, the annual parasite incidence from 2000 to 2016 and the number of malaria cases from 2010 to 2020 in the Yunnan border area, China. The six major phases of malaria from hyperendemicity to elimination program are indicated by the arrows.

with malaria outbreak. The "three mass measures," namely, indoor residual spraying with insecticides, mass drag administration for preventive treatment and radical cure treatment, were carried out in the villages with malaria outbreaks (Li et al., 2017; Wang and Yang, 2013). To ensure adherence of mass drag administration, health workers visited each household every day to conduct directly observe therapy for malaria prevention and radical cure treatment (Xu et al., 2021a,b). In 1977, the number of malaria cases was reduced to a total of 19,505 cases and the annual malaria incidence dropped to 5.9 per 1000 person-years (Fig. 3). The intensive interventions successfully controlled the malaria resurgence and epidemic (Wang and Yang, 2013; Xu et al., 2017).

3.4 Consolidating and scaling up achievement, 1978–2002

3.4.1 Challenges faced

The malaria resurgence and epidemic were effectively controlled, and the annual malaria incidence was decreased to 4.3 per 1000 person-years in the border area in 1978 (Fig. 3). With the policy of "Reform and Open Door" to stimulate economic activities, the public health was facing more challenges than ever before. First, prior to 1978, the primary health care service system comprised of three levels of county health facilities including anti-epidemic stations, township hospitals and village health stations. The primary health care service system in rural areas was called the rural cooperative medical system that was developed under collective financing and public support from the People's Commune. "Barefoot doctors" (community health workers) were the backbone of the rural cooperative medical system and their mission was emphasized in public health. The rural cooperative medical system which was operated by the villagers on a collective and mutual aid basis effectively maintained activities of malaria prevention and treatment. The villagers received free medical care in the rural cooperative medical system (Taylor, 1981). With reform of economic system in rural area, the rural cooperative medical system lost collective financing and public support from the People's Commune. Operation of the medical system largely depended on marketing mechanism under the policy of "Reform and Open Door." The public health received less attention from the governments. Some of health staff, including community health workers, left the village health stations for better economic income in private medication sector (Hsiao, 1984; Shi, 1993). The number and percentage of under-reported malaria cases was gradually increasing due to the reduced sensitivity of malaria surveillance system). Fig. 3 shows a decreasing trend of the annual malaria incidence in the border areas from 1978 to 2002. However, the increased number and frequency of malaria outbreaks underlined that the malaria situation might not be true (Wang and Yang, 2013). In 1987, a malaria epidemic with five malaria-related deaths occurred, and the annual malaria incidence increased to 34.41 per 1000 person-years in Hekou County on the China–Vietnam border (Hekou Center for Diseases Control and Prevention, 2015; Xu et al., 2017). In 1989 alone, there were 39 villages with malaria outbreaks, 42.9% (379/883) of slide positive rate and 33.3% (126/379) *P. falciparum* malaria among the population with outbreaks (Xu and Liu, 1997). Second, internal and transnational population migration increased transmission and the spread of malaria. It was estimated from the departments of public security, customs and frontier inspection that there were more than 10 million mobile people in the Yunnan border area. There were four million entries by foreigners and 2.5 million re-entries by Chinese nationals each year. Internal and cross border migrants had a high morbidity and mortality. Most parts of the border areas with tropical or subtropical climate, development of the tropical agriculture attracted a large amount of migrant farm workers who were usually from inland non-malarious areas and lacking immunity to malaria, and then suffered malaria seriously when they stayed in the border area (Wang and Yang, 2013). An active detection conducted in 1990 reported 60.1% of parasite prevalence (43.1% *P. falciparum*) and 9.9% of mortality at Jiabuto rubber plantation in Mengla County on the China-Myanmar-Lao border. In 1991, among about 40,000 lumber workers returned to Yunnan from Myanmar, 22.7% of them had malaria (Wang and Yang, 2013). In 1992, nearly 1000 farm workers returned to Yunnan Tengchong County from Myanmar, with a 34.02% parasite prevalence rate, 26.6% *P. falciparum* including two deaths (Zhang et al., 1996). In 1995, the average parasite rate of fever cases was 6.7% (580/8694) with 1.8% *P. falciparum* among migrant workers returning from neighbouring countries in Yunnan (Xu and Liu, 1997). Third, insurgency and conflict within Myanmar led to an influx of refugees, often bringing malaria with them. In 1987 alone, a total of 7838 refugees entered 45 villages in the Yunnan border area leading to malaria outbreak, increasing the annual malaria incidence in Longchuan County from 0.52 per 1000 person-years in 1985 to 4.57 per 1000 person-years in 1989 (Xu and Liu, 1997). Fourth, there were 13 indigenous ethnic minorities living in the Yunnan border area. In spite of lacking data in detail across the Yunnan border area, results of cross-sectional studies reported indigenous ethnic minorities with higher malaria burden, 30.5% (12.4% *P. falciparum*) of parasite prevalence at a Hani ethnicity village, 12.5% (2.5% *P. falciparum)* at a Dai ethnicity village and 14.3% (4.8% *P. falciparum*) at a Wa ethnicity village in 1990s (Xu and Liu, 1997).

3.4.2 Control strategy and achievement

Phase 1978–2002 was really a challenging era to the public health in China. The focus of governmental mission was economic development. Marketing mechanism was used in the health service including the public health. The public health was also operated using marketing mechanism (Hsiao, 1984; Shi, 1993). Due to availability of a lot of malaria patients, diagnosis and treatment for malaria was one of the main economic income channels for health facilities including the public health sector. In the other hand, the local governments at each level could only provide budgets for human resources of the public health, and the higher level of the health authorities was lacking of funding to invest in the public health (Hsiao, 1984; Shi, 1993). In the context of lacking budgets for the public health, the higher level of the governments still requested the public health sector and the local governments to gradually reduce malaria burden on the basis of maintaining a stable malaria situation. In order to meet the governmental goal, the anti-epidemic stations had to make money through providing health and technical services including diagnosis and treatment for malaria. A part of the economic income from the health and technical services were used to award the bonuses and welfare for their staff. Another part of the economic income was used to procure antimalarial drugs, insecticides and equipment to prepare responding to any possible malaria outbreaks. In term of this operation, the anti-epidemic station is really a suitable name for its mission fighting outbreaks of infectious diseases (Wang and Yang, 2013).

The more malaria patients, the more choices to make money, this kind of public health service operation was actually difficult to control malaria effectively in the Yunnan border area. Some private clinics even regardless of the national guidelines for malaria treatment administered sub-treatment therapies for malaria patients to keep the money-making sources. Some public health staff often commented "the more work done, the more malaria cases detected." To solve the challenge faced and to fight malaria effectively, the Yunnan Health Department and the Yunnan Institute of Malaria Control (the former Yunnan Institute of Parasitic Diseases) conceived and carried out the joint malaria control program in the Yunnan border area from 1988 to 1997. A provincial project office was established in the YIPD to provide technical supports and to coordinate cross prefecture activities, including developing the protocol of border malaria control, terms of reference, annul work plan, and organizing annual monitoring and evaluation (ME). Eight border prefectures were organized into three joint adventure groups, namely, Western Yunnan Group consisting of Nujiang, Baoshan and Dehong Prefectures; Southern Yunnan Group consisting of Lincang, Puer and Xishuangbanna Prefectures; Southeastern Yunnan Group consisting of Honghe and Wenshan Prefectures. The YIPD funded itself and each prefecture funded itself. Every prefecture chaired and coordinated activities within a joint adventure group in turn each year conducting cross prefecture ME activities and sharing experiences (Wang and Yang, 2013). The technical strategy of "one village, one strategy" was developed to control malaria. This strategy categorized all natural villages into four stratifications each year dynamically based on their annual malaria incidence in the last 3 years. Targeted interventions should be carried out in each village according to its type (Table 1) (Xu et al., 1998).

Table 1 Malaria area stratification and interventions in the Yunnan border area.

Tier	definition	Interventions
Type 1	A village with annual parasite incidence (API) $\geq$1%, or malaria clinical attack rate $\geq$ 10% last year	(1) Mass drug administration for radical cure in December–February next year and preventive treatment in May–October; (2) Presumptive treatment of all febrile patients for malaria; (3) Two rounds of indoor residual spraying (IRS) or dipping bed nets with pyrethroid insecticides
Type 2	A village with API <1%, or malaria clinical attack rate < 10% last year, but there are indigenous cases in the last 3 years	(1) Radical cure treatment of people with malaria attack history in last 2 years; (2) Presumptive treatment of suspected malaria cases and febrile patients without clear causes for malaria (3) One rounds of IRS or dipping bed nets with pyrethroid insecticides
Type 3	A village without indigenous cases, only imported cases in the last 3 years	(1) Radical cure treatment of people with malaria attack history in last 2 years; (2) Presumptive treatment of suspected malaria cases and febrile patients without clear causes for malaria; (3) IRS with pyrethroid insecticides in houses of malaria patients and neighbours
Type 4	A village without any malaria cases in the last 3 years	

Despite this natural village-based stratification and interventions were unable to fully carry out due to the shortage of financial investment and other resources. The joint malaria control program timely provided advocacies to the local government paying attention to malaria control at the same time of economic development. This approach basically maintained a stable malaria situation in the context of "Reform and Open Door" (Wang and Yang, 2013). Phase 1978–2002 was also an innovative time of malaria control in Yunnan. Under the governmental requirement of reducing malaria incidence year after year, the public health facilities, from YIPD, anti-epidemic stations at the prefecture and county levels, and even some township hospitals, designed and carried out a lot of malaria intervention trials or operational researches based on their localities. The experiences obtained were used and scaled up to control malaria in their local contexts (Xu et al., 2021a,b). Fig. 4 shows the intervention acctivities in phase 1978–2002.

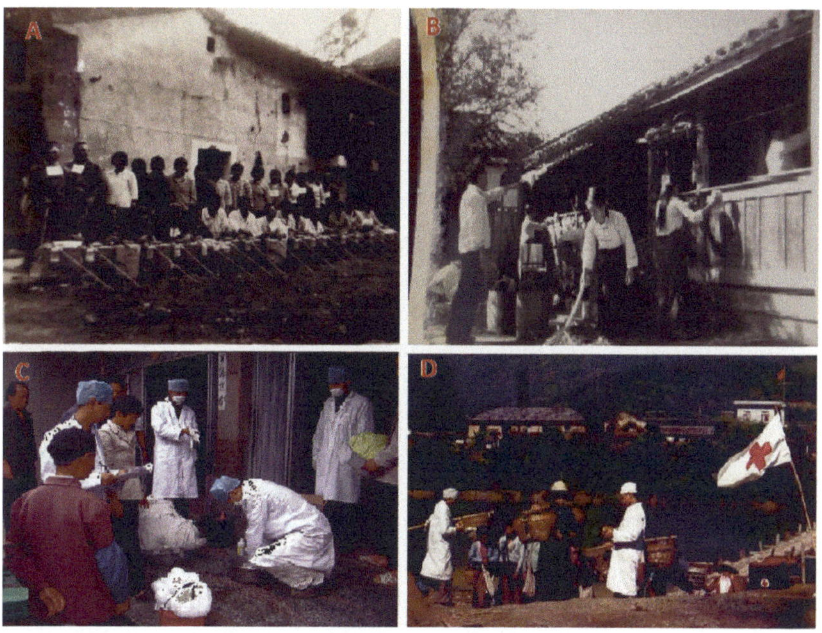

Fig. 4 Working pictures in the Yunnan border area during 1978–2002: (A) A community team of indoor residual spraying (IRS); (B) Mobilizing community to clean houses and environment prior to IRS; (C) Dipping bed nets with insecticides for villagers; (D) Administering antimalarial drugs to border crossers for prophylaxis.

3.4.3 Adverse impact

In the background of lacking financial investment in malaria control activities and of that the governments could mainly pay for the salary of the public health staff, the malaria situation was relatively stable in the Yunnan border area, and the reported malaria incidence was decreased in general (Fig. 3). However, the marketing mechanism could not solve the public health problem. A high proportion of malaria cases was underreported in the reporting system of malaria information because of two reasons. First, lacking of the governmental supervision to the report of malaria cases, the private medical facilities did not usually report malaria cases that they diagnosed. Second, some of the local governments at the county and township levels might not encourage their public health facilities to report malaria cases that they detected. In 2002, a survey of underreported malaria cases found that the underreported rate on average of malaria cases was as high as 88.8% based on the history of malaria attacks among a sample of 30,580 people in Yunnan. The underreported rates of malaria cases in the border counties were higher than the mean rate of the whole province, such as Mengla 90.1%, Menglian 97.8%, Longling 95.5% and Lancang 95.9%. Based on the survey of underreported malaria cases, it was estimated that there were approximately 100 thousand malaria cases in the Yunnan border area in 2003 (Zhang et al., 2004).

3.5 Malaria from control to pre-elimination, 2003–2013

In January 2003, the first round of the Global Fund to fight AIDS, Tuberculosis and Malaria (GFATM) with a malaria control program was rolled out in the 25 border counties. With an improvement in the laboratory diagnosis and the reduced underreported malaria cases, a total of 10,349 confirmed malaria cases and 17.6 per 10,000 person-years of API were reported in the Yunnan Border area in 2003. The GFATM malaria program helped solving the problem of financial shortage in equipment, supplies and control activities. The natural village-based stratification and intervention were able to continuously and fully implement from 2003 to 2013. The API was reduced to 13.5 per 10,000 person-years in 2006, followed by 2.3 per 10,000 person-years in 2010 and 0.6 per 10,000 person-years in 2013 (Fig. 3). The significant reduction in malaria burden made it possible to completely switch the malaria program from control to elimination across the Yunnan border area. As one of the WHO's recommendations, the malaria program with the API <1.0 per 1000 person-years, equal to less than

100 new cases per year in a district with a population of 100,000 people, can started the phase of malaria elimination (WHO, 2014). In China, the smallest unit for elimination was a county, and most counties have a population of over one million. The API >1 per 10,000 person-years was considered stilling being in the phase of pre-elimination. In another word, the national malaria elimination program recommended that the elimination phase was initiated after achieving an API < 1 per 10,000 person-years. The action plan of China malaria elimination (2010–2020) rolled out in July 2010. The county-based stratification and intervention for malaria elimination were carried out for malaria detection and response following the national requirement in Yunnan. The strategy of malaria elimination is an individual malaria case-based detection and response. Because of the malaria situation and complex ecology in the Yunnan border area, the population-based control strategy had to still be used to decrease the malaria incidence from 2010 to 2013.

China and Myanmar signed "The agreement of cross border malaria control" on June 7, 2005 (China and Myanmar, 2005). With Supports from the International Collaboration Department of National Ministry of Health (the National Health Commission at present) in China, Yunnan has carried out "The joint malaria control project along China–Myanmar Border" since 2005 (Zhou et al., 2015). Under the agreement framework, YIPD and Health Poverty Action (HPA, formerly, Health Unlimited) that is a UK-based nongovernment organization successfully applied for and implemented the sixth and tenth rounds of GFATM malaria projects along the China-Myanmar border from 2007 to 2013. The two GFATM malaria projects obtained a total budget of US$ 32,512,550. China allocated a total of US$ 17,196,071 (52.9%) to the HPA for malaria control activities in the border areas of Myanmar. When cars, drugs, bed nets and other equipment were included, more than 70% of the two grants received by China center for disease control and prevention (CDC) were used in Myanmar. A large amount of interventions successfully reduced the malaria burden by 90% in the five Special Regions of Myanmar, decreasing malaria parasite prevalence from 13.6% (95% CI, 12.7–14.6%) in March 2008, to 1.5% (95% CI, 1.2–2.0%) in November 2013. The main hyperendemic areas in Myanmar's border areas were reduced to only three main malaria hot spots by 2013, namely, Laiza and nearby areas in Kachin Special Region II (KR2), Salween River Valley in Shan Special Region II and Small Golden Triangle in Shan Special Region IV. The malaria burden was reduced by 95% in 19 China's counties bordering Myanamr, decreasing the API from 19.6 per 10,000 person-years in 2006 to 0.9 per 10,000 person-years in 2013. The dramatically reduced malaria burden along the China-Myanmar border contributed to the success of malaria elimination in China (Xu et al., 2016, 2021a,b).

3.6 Malaria elimination 2014–16

Yunnan's 104 inland counties kept pace with the whole country to start malaria elimination action since July 2010. With high political commitment, the malaria elimination was put into the government's work goals at each level (Yang et al., 2022). The Malaria elimination requires full surveillance of malaria cases and rapid response to malaria foci (WHO, 2014; Xu et al., 2021a,b). According to the "1-3-7" approaches, report of malaria cases within 1 day, confirmation and investigation of malaria cases within 3 days, and an appropriate public health response to prevent further transmission within 7 days (Cao et al., 2014) and "The protocol of Yunnan malaria elimination action plan (2010–2020)," the Yunnan border area began to completely carried out the intensive surveillance and the rapid individual case-based response for the malaria elimination in January 1, 2014. The date was later than the national malaria elimination action starting date, July 1, 2010 (YHD, 2010). A total of 481,772 febrile patents were tested by microscopy or RDTS for malaria in the border area from 2014 to 2016. The elimination interventions, including individual and focused epidemiological investigations and public health responses, were conducted on all 1240 malaria cases in the Yunnan border areas during 2014–2016. Strengthened malaria surveillance ensured the timely detection of parasite infections and rapid response to prevent further transmission. The transmission of *P. falciparum* and *P. vivax* malaria was successfully interrupted in the Yunnan border areas since May 2015, and April 2016, respectively (Zhao et al., 2020).

3.7 Preventing reintroduction and certificating malaria free 2017–June 2021

Despite the malaria transmission was interrupted in the Yunnan border areas, Yunnan borders three malaria endemic countries. Imported malaria can be caused by both border crossers and parasite-infected *Anopheles* mosquitoes, which fly over the boundary from endemic areas of neighbour countries. The threat from Vietnam and Lao PDR is slight. Vietnam reported that the malaria transmission was interrupted in its northern provinces bordering

China (Thanh et al., 2015). Laos also reported a rapid progress towards localized elimination goal in its northern provinces bordering China (Kounnavong et al., 2017). The Yunnan border area first achieved malaria free status for at least 3 years in two prefectures along China-Vietnam border, Honghe Prefectures in 2015 (Xu et al., 2017), and then Wenshan Prefectures in 2016 (Yang et al., 2022). To prevent the reintroduction of malaria transmission effectively, Yunnan further categorized 25 border counties into three tiers (types A, B and C) based on the malaria hyperendemicity in border area of neighbouring countries and the specificity of 25 border counties in 2017, namely 12 type A counties, seven type B counties, and six type C counties. The type C counties only border Vietnam, and did not need additional investment for special interventions. The type B counties needed to strengthen malaria case surveillance. The type A counties needed special interventions and more investment of human and financial resources. *Anopheles* mosquito mark-release-recapture experiments around the world estimated that the mean distance travelled of female *Anopheles* was not more than 2.5 km (Guerra et al., 2014). According to the comprehensive assessment of the vulnerability and receptivity on each border community in China and the malaria endemicity within 2.5 km-wide perimeter border areas in Myanmar, 16 natural villages were considered still being in the threat of border-spill malaria in 2018. Border-spill malaria is defined as a kind of imported malaria that is caused by parasite-infected *Anopheles* from the border endemic areas of neighbour countries. Integrated interventions, including proactive and passive detection of malaria parasites, enhancement and optimization of vector surveillance, further strengthening of timely detection with high-quality confirmed diagnosis and prompt action based on the surveillance results were conducted in these 16 natural villages with a high risk of malaria reintroduction (Xu et al., 2021a,b). That intensive interventions successfully prevented the reintroduction of malaria transmission in the Yunnan border area made sure timely national malaria elimination certification in June 2020 and WHO malaria free certification in June 2021.

4. Experiences

Malaria from hyperendemicity to elimination in the Yunnan border area is a complex process of more than seven decades. In every phase of the process, Yunnan was based on the locality, including malaria burden, governing system, health service structure, socioeconomic development and ecology to innovate approaches for malaria control and elimination. The following experiences can be obtained from this case study.

4.1 High political commitment

A high political commitment is input in every one of six phases from the beginning of malaria control to elimination at different level. At the beginning of the founding of P. R. China, governments mobilized as much as possible financial and human resources to establish the primary care system carrying out malaria control in the Yunnan border area. In the context of mainly assuring human resource and lacking of governmental budget for malaria control interventions during 1978–2002, the governmental policy was still to require the public health sector reducing malaria incidence every year through encouraging innovations for malaria control. The high political commitment pushed the public health sector managing to use market mechanism to raise fund for malaria control activities, meanwhile, the public health sector conducted innovate intervention trials or operational researches to develop cost-effective strategies based on its own locality. At every level, the malaria elimination was one of the governmental work objectives and so was in the governmental working agenda during 2010–20.

4.2 Updated strategy in each phase of the malaria program

Innovation is always on the way. Technical strategies and measures have continuously been updated in malaria control and elimination in the border area. A "locality oriented, malaria burden oriented, special strategy for special area and special time" principle was conducted to encouraging every border county innovating approaches of malaria control and elimination. According to this principle, the Yunnan border counties continuously developed new intervention approaches based on its own locality, including malaria burden (incidence and prevalence), risk level of malaria infection, local socioeconomic conditions and ecology. From 1956 to 1960, the "three mass measures," namely, MDA for radical cure treatment, MDA for preventive treatment and mass IRS with insecticides were widespread used to reduce malaria burden during the first 5-year provincial malaria control program. From 1961 to 1970, the second and the third provincial 5-year malaria control program first categorized the whole province into three tiers (high, moderate and low) of malaria endemic areas based on annual incidence. The "three mass measures" was continuously conducted to reduce malaria incidence in the high malaria endemic areas. In the moderate and low malaria endemic areas, strategies were to eliminate parasite reservoirs first, including standardized treatment of clinical patients and parasite carriers in time, and radical cure treatment for people who had malaria an attack history last year in the low malaria transmitting season. The IRS with insecticides was only carried out in villages with potential transmission. The preventive treatment was only administered to the people with a high risk of malaria infection, such as people who went to foot hill for agriculture production in river valley areas (Wang and Yang, 2013; Zhou et al., 2022). From 1988 to 2009, all natural villages were categorized into four stratifications each year dynamically based on malaria incidence in the last 3 years. Different approaches of interventions were conducted according to the natural village-based stratification (Xu et al., 1998). This "one village, one strategy" strategy made interventions more targeted and cost-effective. The strategy is consisted with the WHO's recommendation that the stratification is initially performed at the lowest geographical level for which operational decisions can be made (WHO, 2014). From 2010 forward, intensive surveillance and rapid response to any possible malaria cases was used to clear parasite reservoirs and interrupt malaria transmission. Additionally, the widespread application of new pyrethroid insecticides, artemisinins and its derivatives, other highly effective antimalarial drugs such as pyronaridine and artemisinin-based combination therapy significantly improved efficacy of the malaria control interventions after the later 1980s (Yang et al., 2022).

4.3 Innovative malaria treatment schemes in the malaria program

Drug-based treatment is the primary intervention in malaria control and elimination. Asymptomatic and submicroscopic parasite density (especially for *P. vivax*) together with the limitations of microscopist ability and rapid diagnostic tests may lead to underdetection or misdiagnosis. From 2008 to 2016, three targeted treatment programs were undertaken in the KR2, Myanmar. Program I (2008–11) that was supported by the sixth round of GFATM malaria project treated all confirmed, clinical and suspected cases; program II (2012 – 13) that was supported by the 10th round of GFATM malaria project treated confirmed and clinical cases; and program III (2014–16) that was supported by the Myanmar's Global Fund New Funding Model to Intensify Malaria Control Project only treated confirmed cases. During program I (2008–11), malaria burden was reduced by 61%

(95% CI: 58%–74%) and the actual API decreased from 9.8 (95% CI: 9.6–10.1) per 100 person-years in 2008 to 3.8 (3.6–4.1) per 100 person-years in 2011. Amid program II (2012–13), the malaria burden increased by 33% (95% CI: 22%–46%) and the actual API increased from 2.1 (95% CI: 2.0–2.3) per 100 person-years in 2012 to 2.8 (95% CI: 2.7–2.9) per 100 person-years in 2013. During program III (2014–16) the malaria burden increased furtherly by 60% (95%CI: 51–69%) and the actual API increased from 3.2 (95% CI: 3.0–3.3) per 100 person-years in 2014 to 5.1 (95% CI: 4.9–5.2) per 100 person-years in 2016 (Liu et al., 2018a,b). The experiences of the Myanmar KR2 and the experiences of transition of radical, preventive and presumptive treatment regimens for malaria in China (Xu et al., 2021a,b) indicate MDA can rapidly reduce the malaria burden in hyperendemic areas; however, it might not be necessary for mesoendemic situations. In the mesoendemic areas, treatment for all confirmed, clinical and suspected cases, not just targeting confirmed malaria cases, combined with vector controls might be necessary. In the hyperendemic areas with intensive transmission, MDA can effectively clear parasite reservoirs; meanwhile, vector control should be considered as an important supplementary intervention too.

4.4 Improved information system supports surveillance and response to malaria

Unique natural geography and location create a complex ecological system with hills, gorges and snowy mountains in the Yunnan border area. The elevation ranges from 76.4 m on the China-Vietnam border in the southern Yunnan to 6740 on the China-Myanmar border in the northwestern Yunnan. Diversity of the landforms makes difficulty of transportation and communication. A promptly accurate reporting system of malaria information is needed for rapid responses to any suspected malaria cases. However, the Yunnan border area mainly used a paper-based record and report information system prior to the establishment of China Information System for Disease Control and Prevention (CISDCP). The provincial level could routinely collect malaria information once a year. A sample survey on the underreported malaria indicated more than 90% of malaria cases were underreported in the Yunnan border area in 2002 (Zhang et al., 2004). Problems in malaria surveillance and information reporting system might be one cause of seriously underreported malaria cases prior to 2003. The delayed reports of malaria information might lead to inappropriate response or postpone the response. The CISDCP that reports malaria cases in real time began to cover all Yunnan's counties since 2008.

The CISDCP makes sure the complete implementation of the "1-3-7" response approaches and the work of malaria diagnostic reference laboratory network during malaria elimination phase.

4.5 Engagement of the broader communities

Engagement of the broader communities reduced the amount of governmental budget and achieved a high coverage of interventions. When malaria control activities needed the participation of communities, the local governmental officers at township and village level helped out to notify communities through public education programs on malaria and mobilize community involvement. Under technical support of health staff, communities assigned human resources to conduct IRS with insecticides, and work as guides in drug administration for radical and preventive treatment prior to 2003. Village health workers (VHW) and village malaria control workers (VMCW) were assigned to involve in the drug administration (Xu et al., 2017; Yang and Zhou, 2015). House-to-house visits every day conducting to directly observe therapy was the core to this methodology for increasing coverage, compliance and safety in MDA (Li and Wei, 1993; Xu et al., 2017). In the daily house visits, the VHW or VMCW questioned individuals about adverse effects of the treatment taken the previous day; and then the VHW or VMCW would made a decision on whether the next dose should be given. In the case of there was an adverse effect reported, such as black tea coloured urine after primaquine administration in people with glucose-6-phosphate dehydrogenase deficiency, treatment would be stopped immediately. According to the national guidelines and to the type of adverse reaction and severity of clinical symptoms, a proper rescue treatment was followed (Xu et al., 2021a,b). To those with minor symptoms such as low grade haemoglobinuria, primaquine would be discontinue dosing, while those showing more severe adverse effects would be given a blood transfusion. This method made sure a sound coverage and safety of the treatment interventions (NHFPC, 2016; Xu et al., 2017; Yang and Zhou, 2015). In a word, broader community engagement is not just able to increase human resources, and also help to improve coverage, cost-effectiveness and the safety of control interventions (Xu et al., 2021a,b).

4.6 Cross-border collaboration and communication

Cross border collaboration and communication ensured the successful application and implementation of the 6th and 10th rounds of the Global Fund to fight AIDS, Tuberculosis and Malaria (GFATM) with two malaria projects along the China-Myanmar border from 2007 to 2013. Interventions of the two GFATM malaria projects created a prerequisite for malaria elimination by the dramatically reduced malaria incidence along the China-Myanmar border (Xu et al., 2016). In June of 2014, an outbreak of *P. falciparum* malaria caused by imported malaria from the Salween River Valley hot spot (Liu et al., 2018a,b; Xu et al., 2021a,b) was reported in the Shan Special Region II of Myanmar. Despite the outbreak site (a rubber plantation) was about 10 km away from the China-Myanmar border, most of people in the plantation were the Lahu ethnic minority who immigrated into Myanmar from China. China and Myanmar collaboratively controlled the outbreak and prevented malaria exportation to China (Liu et al., 2016) (Fig. 5).

Due to military conflict in the Kachin State of Myanmar led to less cross-border collaboration and communication with the Special Region II (KR2) from 2014 to 2016. The reduced collaboration and communication led to malaria resurgence (Liu et al., 2018a,b) after the successful implementation of the two GFATM malaria projects in the KR2 of Myanmar (Xu et al., 2016). The Laiza and nearby areas with a population of approximately 30,000 people reported 2080 malaria cases in 2016. To reduce the imported malaria threat from the Laiza and nearby areas, the YIPD and Yingjiang County CDC provided necessary antimalarial drugs, insecticides and other supplies to the KR2, meanwhile, sent a technical team to station in Laiza providing technical assistance. The strengthened collaboration and effective interventions reduced the number of malaria cases reported in the Laiza and nearby areas from 1936 cases in 2017 followed by 664 cases in 2018 and then 274 cases in 2019. Correspondingly, the number of imported malaria cases in Yingjiang County reduced from 179 cases in 2017 followed by 106 cases in 2018, and then 92 cases in 2019 and 75 cases in 2020. In a word, cross border collaboration and communication is important for malaria control and elimination in the border area, especially for preventing malaria to spill over the boundary by parasite- infected female anopheline mosquitoes (Xu et al., 2021a,b).

4.7 Interaction between control effectiveness and socioeconomic development

Malaria control and socioeconomic development interacted with each other. The controlled malaria promoted the socioeconomic development (Fig. 1), and the socioeconomic development created conditions for the malaria elimination. In terms of socioeconomic development for malaria

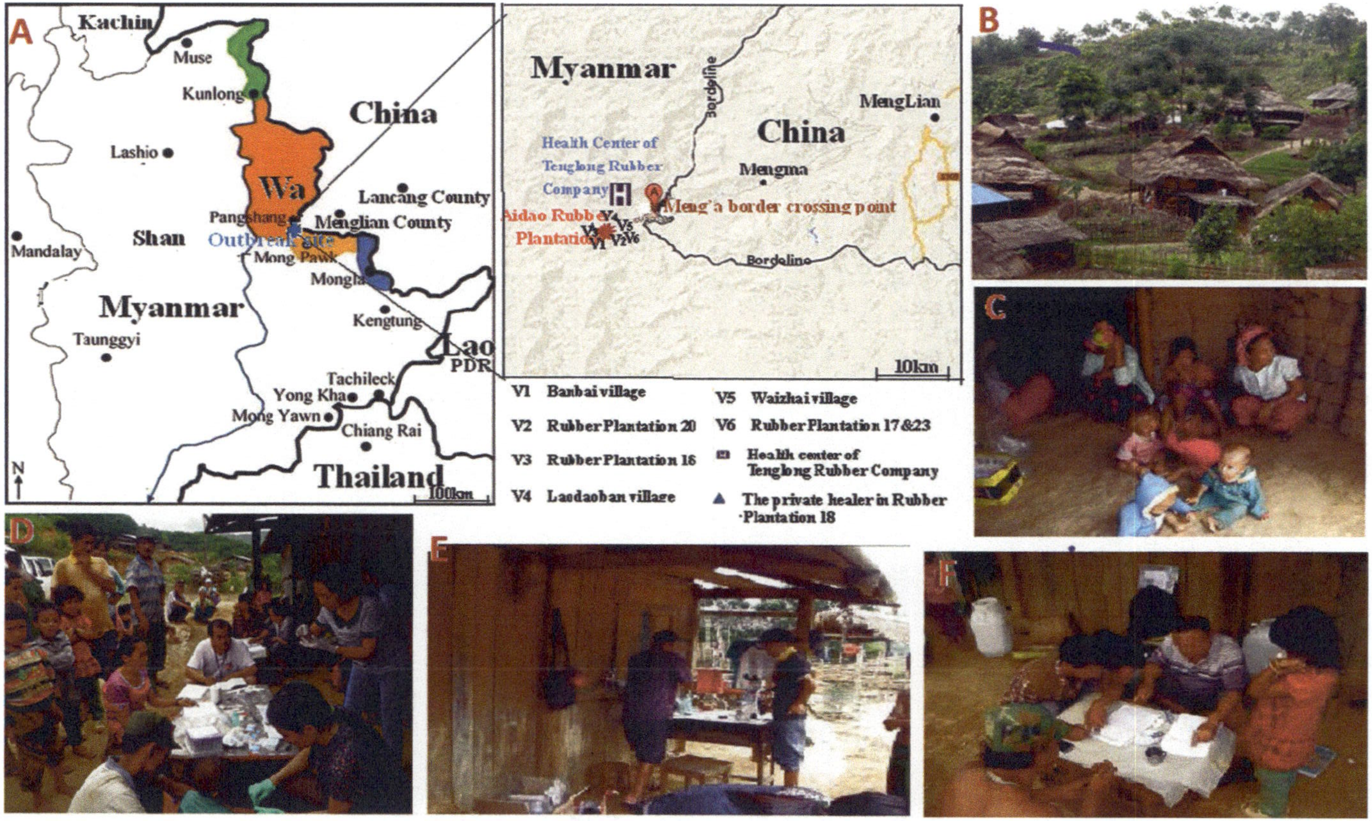

Fig. 5 Pictures showing the China-Myanmar collaborative response to an outbreak of *P. falciparum* malaria in the Shan Special Region II of Myanmar in June 2014: (A) Location map of the outbreak site and nearby areas; (B–C) Living houses and people; (D–F) Diagnosis and treatment people with malaria infection, from preparing blood smear to microscopy followed by administrating antimalarial drugs (Liu et al., 2016).

control and elimination, the website-based CISDCP that reported malaria in real time is one of socioeconomic development outcomes. Particularly, the malaria hyperendemic areas are always in remote areas in Yunnan. Most of the malaria hyperendemic areas had no roads for cars in the Yunnan border area in 1950s. The health workers had to walk and use horses carrying equimpment, insecticids and other supplies into the hyperendemic areas. They had to travel for more than 1 month from Kunming (Yunnan Provincial Capital) to the hyperendemic area along the international borders. Till 1990s, the staff of some county anti-epidemic stations needed walk for 3 days from their county capital towns to some remote border villages carrying out malaria control activities. The road construction has always been one of the priorities in China. The transportation is no longer a problem today. The health workers can drive their cars to any villages. A family owns at least one motorcycle, and most families own their cars. Most villagers drive their own motorcycles or cars to the township hospitals (the health centers) for the malaria laboratory test and treatment is now within less than 30 min (Xu et al., 2017). The improvement of transportation and information system makes sure detecting and reporting malaria cases in time, and then conducting appropriate public health responses following the "1-3-7" requirement.

5. Lessons

Five lessons can be learned from the historical review of malaria from hyperendemicity to elimination in the Yunnan border area.

5.1 The sustainability of the malaria control program needs a political stability

Because of the urgent request from more than 40 famous men in Simao City, Dr Hou came back to his hometown from the Yunnan Military Hospital in Kunming fighting the malaria epidemic (Fig. 1) in 1935. He established the Simao-Puer Hospital to treat malaria, and made the mosquito figure lanterns by himself to deliver knowledge of malaria, its vector, transmission and control. However, he had to return to Kunming in November in the same year because the Simao-Puer Hospital lacked funding paying for its staff work (Zhou et al., 2022). In 1942, the malaria control activities in Yunnan had to be abandoned because Japanese Army occupied the south and the west of Yunnan Province (Wang and Yang, 2013). From May 1966 to early 1970, people including health personnel spent more time involving in political activities. The reduced malaria control intensity led to the malaria resurgence in Yunnan again (Wang and Yang, 2013; Xu et al., 2017). The continuous military conflicts now days in the northern Myanmar still challenge malaria control along China-Myanmar border and preventing malaria reintroduction in China. All these events indicate the importance of a stable political situation for malaria control in anywhere of the world.

5.2 The malaria control and elimination needs multi-sector collaboration

There still was a high political will for malaria control in Yunnan during 1978–2002. The high-level governments requested the low-level governments and the public health sector to maintain the malaria stability and to reduce the malaria incidence every year in spite of lacking budget for malaria control activities. Paying less attention to malaria case surveillance and reports appeared to be one of the simplest solutions for the low-level governments to meet the requirement of the high-level governments. Under the market mechanism of public health services, malaria diagnosis and treatment itself was a channel of making money. In this context, the public health services paid more attention to the malaria treatment but less to the malaria prevention. The reduced sensitivity of malaria surveillance led to significantly underreported malaria cases (Zhang et al., 2004). This lesson documents that the marketing mechanism cannot solve the public health problems, including malaria control. Learnt from this lesson, the action plan of China malaria elimination (2010–20) was formulated and released by a total of 13 departments including the Ministry of Health, the development and Reform Commission and the Ministry of Finance, etc. Following the national model and instruction, the local protocols of malaria elimination action plan (2010–20) in Yunnan, from the provincial level to the county level, were also formulated and released by the corresponding sectors. In the Yunnan border area, each sector played its capacity and contributed malaria elimination in their localities.

5.3 The reduction of malaria burden in border areas of neighbour countries needs cross-border collaboration at the local level

To reduce the risk of malaria reintroduction, a malaria elimination program needs to collaborate with countries which export malaria (WHO, 2014). In many setting, the two central governments might have agreed the cross border malaria control collaboration between two countries, implementation of the agreed activities might still remain a big challenge (Xu et al., 2021a,b; Zhou et al., 2015). The complex administration system might slow down the implementation of the agreed activities or even make the implementation impossible. The reduction of cross border collaboration and communication might increase malaria incidence in the border area of neighbour countries, and then increase imported malaria in the Yunnan border area. To simplify the process and overcome barriers caused by different administrative systems in cross border malaria control, the two central governments can decide on an agreed framework and empower corresponding local government agencies along with civil society organizations to carry out activities with mutual benefit along the common border areas (Xu et al., 2021a,b). From 2013 to 2016, the API increased from 2.8 (95% CI: 2.7–2.9) per 100 person-years in 2013 to 5.1 (95% CI: 4.9–5.2) per 100 person-years in 2016 in Myanmar KR2. One of reasons for the malaria resurgence was the reduction of collaboration and communication between Myanmar KR2 and the Yunnan border area (Liu et al., 2018a,b). The increased incidence in the Myanmar KR2 led to more imported malaria cases in China Yingjiang County bordering Myanmar KR2, from 48 cases in 2013 to 96 cases in 2016.

5.4 The effective malaria control and elimination program need prompt finding and rapid responses to malaria foci

Accurate information of malaria epidemiology is the basis of scientifically decision-making and investment of the stockholders for malaria control and elimination (Xu et al., 2021a,b). The inaccurate malaria information, especially the underreported malaria cases, might led to the reduced budget from the governments, and then might affect further control activities and efficacy. The lesson of the under reported malaria cases and their adverse impact in Yunnan during 1966–2002 documents that prompt finding and rapidly responding to malaria foci is pivotally important for a malaria control program.

5.5 The sensitivity of surveillance and response system determines the program quality in the elimination stage

In the case that the border area of neighbour countries are still malaria hyperendemic, the border area of malaria elimination country should make sure its malaria surveillance sensitivity and appropriate responses to any possible malaria cases in time. Multisectoral and comprehensive interventions, which include proactive and passive case detection, vector surveillance and evidence-based vector control, are still needed. When vector control measures could not effectively to prevent border-spill malaria caused by parasite-affected anopheline mosquitoes, preventative treatment with anti-malarial drugs might also be needed (Xu et al., 2021a,b).

6. Challenges and recommendations

6.1 Challenges

After the last indigenous malaria case in China was reported from Yingjiang County in the Yunnan border area in April 2016 (Zhao et al., 2020), and even after the WHO certificated China malaria elimination on 30 June 2021 (Burki, 2021), the Yunnan border area is still facing following challenges in preventing reintroduction of malaria transmission.

6.1.1 The threat of imported malaria from neighbour countries will continuously exist for a long term

The Yunnan border area borders Myanmar's five special regions that are out of the central governmental management of Myanmar Union. Some of the five special regions, such as the Kachin Special Region II (KR2) and the Kongkang Autonomous Regions, are still in military conflicts. The health services of ethnic health organizations are too weak to be able to control malaria effectively. The reduced communication and collaboration between China and neighbour countries can increase the risk of reintroduction of malaria transmission. For example, after China's GFATM malaria project was terminated in 2014, the reduced collaborative activities lead to slight malaria resurgences in some border areas of Myanmar since 2014 (Liu et al., 2016, 2018a,b). Particularly, the number of reported malaria cases increased from 518 in 2013 to 2367 in 2016 in KR2's Laiza and nearby areas where are one of the malaria hotspot areas along China-Myanmar border (Xu et al., 2021a,b). The number of imported malaria cases correspondingly increased from 358 in 2013 to 594 cases in 2015 in Yunnan.

6.1.2 The challenge of the COVID-19 pandemic to preventing reintroduction of malaria transmission

The Yunnan border area is also one of the areas facing a high risk of the COVID pandemic in China. To fight the COVID pandemic, some human and financial resources were moved from malaria control to responses to the COVID-19 pandemic. In July 2021, when Yunnan tried to communicate with the Health Authority of Myanmar KR2 to collaborate in rolling back the resurgence of malaria there, the KR2 Department of health answered that they were too busy responding to the COVID-19 pandemic to have human resources fighting malaria. Although the border crossing is strictly limited under the context of the COVID-19 pandemic, the increased malaria incidence in KR2 has led to malaria spilling over the boundary by parasite-infected *Anopheles* mosquitoes into communities in the Yunnan border area. From January to November 2021, Yingjiang County reported a total of 70 cases, and 63 of them were categorized into border-spill malaria cases.

6.1.3 The reduction in vigilance of the local people and the health personnel

The vigilance of the local people and the health personnel, especially the clinical doctors in hospitals, is critical to reduce imported malaria death and prevent reintroduction of malaria transmission in elimination settings (WHO, 2014, 2017). Travellers from malaria endemic countries can always obtain laboratory tests for malaria in time as long as clinical doctors recognize the necessity of testing in China. However, it is a fact that a number of imported malaria deaths are mainly attributable to the delayed diagnosis of malaria because clinical doctors lack vigilance on testing for malaria in China. For example, in November 2021, a Burmese patient with kidney failure was hospitalized in a county hospital in the border area. His resident doctor did not recognize the necessity of malaria testing for more than 3 weeks. The patient had to be moved to a high-level hospital due to his worsened condition, and then the high-level hospital tested him with *Plasmodium malariae*, which was one of the reasons for his kidney failure.

6.1.4 The gradual reduction of political will and commitment

The high political commitment and strong governing system as well as the use of updated technical innovation promised the success of malaria control and elimination in the Yunnan border area. The achievement is attributable to multifactor, including political commitment, socioeconomic development and changing ecological environment as well as effective interventions, and also the complicated interactions between these factors. After reduction of the malaria burden, when the disease is no long one of public health problems in the local governmental schemes, the political will and commitment may normally be decreasing, and then the investment of financial and human sources may gradually being cut down. The reduced investment can challenge preventing reintroduction of malaria transmission in the Yunnan border area.

6.2 Recommendations

6.2.1 Further strengthening cross border collaboration and communication to decrease malaria incidence in the border areas of neighbour countries

China recognized the malaria resurgence in some of Myanmar border areas with China after the end of China's GFATM malaria projects that led to the reduced collaborative activities in malaria control. From 2017 to 2019, China and Myanmar re-strengthened collaborative interventions that reduced the number of malaria cases from 2367 in 2016 to 274 in 2019 again in Laiza and nearby areas, Myanmar KR2 (Xu et al., 2021a,b). The number of imported malaria cases in China Yingjiang County bordering Myanmar KR2 was reduced from 186 in 2016 to 75 in 2020. This promised the WHO malaria elimination certification for China. However, the reduced collaborative interventions due to the COVID-19 pandemic led to malaria resurgence again, and a total of 1532 cases were reported in Laiza and nearby areas of KR2 from January to November 2021. The example of Laiza and nearby areas documents that reduced communication and collaboration may increase malaria incidence in the border areas of neighbour countries and increase the risk of malaria reintroduction in China. In contrast, a reduction in malaria burden in the border area of neighbour countries can help decrease the threat of malaria importation and reestablishment of malaria transmission. To effective reduce the threat of malaria importation, this case study recommends further strengthening cross border collaboration and communication to decrease malaria incidence in the border areas of neighbour countries.

6.2.2 Preparing well to fight the threat of imported malaria in the past COVID pandemic era

The COVID-19 pandemic that limited cross border collaboration and communication for malaria control led to malaria resurgence in some border areas of neighbour countries. Under this context, although the border crossing is strictly limited, the increased malaria incidence in some border areas of neighbour countries leads to malaria spilling over the boundary by parasite-infected *Anopheles* mosquitoes into communities in the Yunnan border area. From January to November 2021, Yingjiang County reported a total of 70 cases, and 63 of them were categorized into border-spill malaria cases. At present, comprehensive intervention, including proactive and passive case detection, vector surveillance, evidence-based vector control and preventative treatment with antimalarial drugs, should be undertaken to prevent border-spill malaria within a 2.5 km-wide perimeter along the boundary in Yunnan (Xu et al., 2021a,b). Meanwhile, this case study also recommends preparing well to fight the threat of imported malaria in the past COVID pandemic era.

6.2.3 Training and retraining health personnel to maintain their vigilance to malaria

The reduction of vigilance and technical capacity in malaria diagnosis and treatment due to rarely seeing malaria patients anymore is one of the challenges to prevent the reintroduction of malaria transmission in elimination settings (Xu et al., 2021a,b). The public health sector must manage to maintain the vigilance of health personnel to malaria, especially of clinical doctors at hospitals, to be able to consider testing malaria in their work. This case study recommends frequently training and retraining health personnel to maintain their vigilance to malaria.

6.2.4 Maintaining the political will and commitment to preventing reintroduction of malaria transmission

Malaria is a continuous public health problem worldwide. There were an estimated 241 million malaria cases in 2020, increased from 227 million in 2019, and malaria deaths increased by 12% compared with 2019, to an estimated 627 thousand (WHO, 2021). Although the WHO certificated malaria free for China, the malaria resurgence in some border areas of neighbour countries increases the risk of malaria reintroduction in the Yunnan border area. This case study recommends that the public health sector should conduct a strong advocacy to the governments for the political will and commitment to preventing reintroduction of malaria transmission.

7. Conclusions

Malaria control and elimination are particular difficult and complex in the Yunnan border area. This achievement is attributed to continuously high political commitment, strategic and technical innovations based on the actual locality, and effective collaboration and communication with neighbour countries to carry out comprehensive cross border interventions. The comprehensive interventions are continuously essential in preventing the reintroduction of malaria transmission in the border area. Access to technical measures requires strong governmental and social support. Other border areas should perform their own operational trials to develop their own effective strategy of malaria control and elimination based on their own local governing system, malaria burden, health service structure, socioeconomic development and ecology.

Acknowledgements

This work was supported by National Natural Science Foundation of P.R. China (Grant no. 81560543 and 81673113).

References

Alonso, P.L., Tanner, M., 2013. Public health challenges and prospects for malaria control and elimination. Nat. Med. 19, 150–155.

Burki, T., 2021. Triumph in China as it is certified malaria-free by WHO. Lancet Inf. Dis. 21, 1220–1221.

Cao, J., Sturrock, H.J.W., Cotter, C., Zhou, S., Zhou, H., et al., 2014. Communicating and monitoring surveillance and response activities for malaria elimination: China's "1-3-7" strategy. PLoS Med. 11 (5), e1001642.

China, M.O.H., Myanmar, M.O.H.S., 2005. The Agreement of Malaria Control in China-Myanmar Border Areas. China ministry of health, Ministry of Health and Sports of Myanma, Kunming. Accessed 9 Jun 2015.

Cui, L., Yan, G., Sattabongkot, J., Cao, Y., Chen, B., Chen, X., et al., 2012. Malaria in the greater Mekong subregion: heterogeneity and complexity. Acta Trop. 121, 227–239.

Dehong Center for Disease Control and Prevention, 2011. Annals of Dehong Center for Disease Control and Prevention. Dehong Center for Disease Control and Prevention, Mangshi.

Department of military history of Academy of Military Sciences, 1991. History of China's Anti Japanese War (Part 2) (in Chinese). PLA Publishing House, Beijing.

Diouf, G., Kpanyen, P.N., Tokpa, A.F., Nie, S., 2014. Changing landscape of malaria in China: progress and feasibility of malaria elimination. Asia Pac. J. Public Health 26, 93–100.

Guerra, A.C., Reiner, J.R.R., Perkins, T.A., Lindsay, S.W., Midega, J.T., Brady, O., et al., 2014. A global assembly of adult female mosquito mark-release-recapture data to inform the control of mosquito-borne pathogens. Parasit. Vectors 7, 276.

Hekou Center for Diseases Control and Prevention, 2015. The Self-Evaluation Report of Malaria Elimination in Hekou County. Hekou Center for Diseases Control and Prevention, Hekou.

Hou, J.X., 1938. A Preliminary Study on the Malaria Epidemic and Investigation at Early Phase of the Epidemic in Simao (in Chinese). vol. 3, The Southwest Frontier, pp. 39–43.

Hsiao, W.C., 1984. Transformation of health care in China. N. Engl. J. Med. 310 (932–6), 26.

Kounnavong, S., Gopinath, D., Hongvanthong, B., Khamkong, C., Sichanthongthip, O., 2017. Malaria elimination in Lao PDR: the challenges associated with population mobility. Infect. Dis. Poverty 6, 81.

Li, X.L., Wei, D.Y., 1993. Efficacy observation of sulfadoxine-pyrimethamine for malaria prophylaxis among border-cross villagers. Chin. J. Parasit. Dis. Con. 6, 158 (in Chinese).

Li, J., Guo, H., Zhang, R., Pu, S., 2017. Malaria transmission, procedures and measures of prevention, control and elimination in Honghe prefecture from 1953 to 2016 (in Chinese). China Trop. Med. 17, 891–894.

Liang, G.S., 1940. Malaria in Simao-Puer area of Yunnan Province and control strategy. Youth Monthly 40, 2.

Liu, H., Xu, J.W., Yang, H.L., Li, M., Sun, C.D., Yin, Y.J., et al., 2016. Investigation and control of a plasmodium falciparum malaria outbreak in Shan special region II of Myanmar along the China-Myanmar border from June to December 2014. Infect. Dis. Poverty 5, 32.

Liu, H., Xu, J.W., Xu, Q.Z., Zeng, Y.R., 2018a. Retrospective analysis of risk factors of slide positivity among febrile patients in the Salween river valley of Shan special region II, northern Myanmar. BMC Public Health 18, 560.

Liu, H., Xu, J.W., Bi, Y., 2018b. Malaria burden and treatment targets in Kachin special region II, Myanmar from 2008 to 2016: a retrospective analysis. PLoS one 13, e0195032.

NHFPC, 2016. Technical Regulations for Antimalarials WS/T 485–2016 (in Chinese). National Health and Family Planning Commission, China, Beijing.

Shi, L., 1993. Health care in China: a rural-urban comparison after the socioeconomic reforms. Bull. World Health Organ. 71, 723–736.

Song, Y.M., 2008. Review of the Epidemic and Control of Infectious Diseases in Yunnan Province During the Period of the republic of China (in Chinese). 15, Transactions of Yunnan Normal University, pp. 48–58.

Tang, L.H., Gao, Q., 2013. Malaria Control and Elimination in China (in Chinese). Shanghai Science and Technical Publisher, Shanghai.

Tang, L.H., Qian, H.L., Xu, S.H., 1991. Malaria and its control in the People's Republic of China. Southeast Asian. J. Trop. Med. Public Health 22, 467–476.

Taylor, R.B., 1981. Primary health care in the People's Republic of China. Postgrad. Med. 70 (69–76), 24.

Thanh, P.V., Hong, N.V., Van, N.V., Malderen, C.V., Obsomer, V., Urgell, A.R., et al., 2015. Epidemiology of forest malaria in Central Vietnam: the hidden parasite reservoir. Malar. J. 14, 86.

Wang, W.R., Yang, H.L., 2013. Yunnan Malaria Control and Research. Yunnan Science and Technology Press, Kunming.

WHO, 2014. Malaria Elimination: A Field Manual for Low and Moderate Endemic Countries. World Health Organization, Geneva (Accessed 20 Feb 2015).

WHO, 2017. A Framework for Malaria Elimination. World Health Organization, Geneva (Accessed 20 Feb 2021).

WHO, 2021. World Malaria Report 2021. World Health Organization, Geneva (Accessed 3 Jan 2022).

Wu, W.H., 1941. General situation of Mengding malaria in Yunnan Province (in Chinese). Chin. J. Med. 27 (8), 483–490.

Xu, J., Liu, H., 1997. Border malaria in Yunnan, China. Southeast Asian J. Trop. Med. Public Health 28, 456–459.

Xu, J., Liu, H., 2012. The challenges of malaria elimination in Yunnan province, People's Republic of China. Southeast Asian J. Trop. Med. Public Health 43, 819–824.

Xu, J.W., Wang, W.R., Xu, S.Y., 1998. Malaria situation and control in border areas and Yuanjiang River basin of Yunnan Province in 1995. Chin. J. Parasit. Dis. Control (in Chinese) 11 (1), 71.

Xu, J.W., Liu, H., Zhang, Y., Guo, X.R., Wang, J.Z., 2015. Risk factors for border malaria in a malaria elimination setting: a retrospective case-control study in Yunnan. China. Am. J. Trop. Med. Hyg. 92, 546–551.

Xu, J.W., Li, Y., Yang, H.L., Zhang, J., Zhang, Z.X., Yang, Y.M., et al., 2016. Malaria control along China-Myanmar border during 2007-2013: an integrated impact evaluation. Infect. Dis. Poverty 5, 75.

Xu, J.W., Li, J.J., Guo, H.P., Pu, S.W., Li, S.M., Wang, R.H., et al., 2017. Malaria from hyperendemicity to elimination in Hekou County on China–Vietnam border: an ecological study. Malar. J. 16, 66.

Xu, J.W., Lee, R., Li, X.H., Liu, H., 2021a. Transition of radical, preventive and presumptive treatment regimens for malaria in China: a systematic review. Malar. J. 20, 10.
Xu, J.W., Lee, R., Lin, Z.R., Zhou, Y.W., Shen, H.M., Zhou, H.N., et al., 2021b. Intensive surveillance, rapid response and border collaboration for malaria elimination: China Yunnan's "3+1" strategy. Malar. J. 20, 396.
Yang, H.L., Zhou, H.N., 2015. Yunnan Malaria (in Chinese). Yunnan Science and Technology Press, Kunming.
Yang, H., Zhou, H., Xu, J., Sun, X., Lin, Z., 2022. Malaria control & elimination in Yunnan, China. Yunnan science and technology press, Kunming (in publication).
Yao, Y.Z., Lin, L.C., Liu, B.R., et al., 1936. Studies on the so-called 'changche' (in Chinese). Chin. J. Med. 22, 2–9.
YHD, 2010. The Protocol of Yunnan Malaria Elimination Action Plan (2010–2020) (in Chinese). Yunnan Health Department, Kunming. Accessed 27 Feb 2019.
Zhang, W., 2005. Regional prejudice and ethnic discrimination: a culture interpretation of Zhangqi and malaria in ancient China (in Chinese). Ethn. Stud. 3, 105–109.
Zhang, Z., Lu, Y., Xu, J., Yin, Z., Yang, Y., et al., 1996. Investigation on malaria prevalence and control in temporary residential areas of collective production returnees. J. Pract. Parasit. Dis. 1, 34.
Zhang, Z.X., Zhou, S., Xu, J.W., Du, Z.W., Chen, G.W., et al., 2004. Investiagtion on missing-report of malaria cases in Yunnan, China (in Chinese). Chin. J. Parasit. Dis. Control 17, 25–27.
Zhao, X., Sun, X., Yang, H., Zhou, D., Yang, J., Guo, T., et al., 2020. A report of the last indigenous malaria case in Yunnan (in Chinese). China Trop. Med. 20, 325–328.
Zheng, Z.Y., 1984. Brief history of major infectious diseases and endemic diseases in Yunnan (in Chinese). In: Historical Materials of Kunming. vol. 3. The Annals of Kunmming Municipality, pp. 172–189.
Zhou, H., Du, L., Yang, H., Zhang, Z., 2015. Innovative Decade of Cross-Border Joint Prevention & Control Project of Malaria and Dengue Fever in Yunnan China-GMS Areas. Yunnan Science and Technology Press, Kunming.
Zhou, H.N., Yang, H.N., Xu, J.W., 2022. Album of malaria from hyperendemicity to elimination in Yunnan. Yunnan Science and Technology Press, Kunming (in publication).

CHAPTER THREE

Surveillance and response systems driving malaria elimination in the mountain areas of Hainan Province

Yuchun Li[a], Shanqing Wang[a], Ximin Hu[a], Yingjuan Huang[b], Renqiang Chen[b], Minchan Lin[c], Huanzhi Xu[c], Rongshen Ye[d], Datian Zhan[e], Shaoling Huang[f], Ji Zhen[g], Xiaodan Wen[h], Guoyi Wang[i], Yong Liu[j], Haishan Li[k], Zaichun Zheng[l], Jian Wang[m], Wen Zeng[a], Feng Meng[a], Xiaoming Huang[a], Guangze Wang[a,*], Bing Yang[a,*], and Yan Chen[a,*]

[a]Hainan Provincial Center for Disease Control & Prevention, Haikou, Hainan, PR China
[b]Sanya City Center for Disease Control & Prevention, Sanya, Hainan, PR China
[c]Wuzhishan City Center for Disease Control & Prevention, Wuzhishan, Hainan, PR China
[d]Baoying County Center for Disease Control & Prevention, Baoying, Jiangsu, PR China
[e]Lingshui County Center for Disease Control & Prevention, Lingshui, Hainan, PR China
[f]Wanning City Center for Disease Control & Prevention, Wanning, Hainan, PR China
[g]Dongfang City Center for Disease Control & Prevention, Dongfang, Hainan, PR China
[h]Danzhou City Center for Disease Control & Prevention, Danzhou, Hainan, PR China
[i]Qiongzhong County Center for Disease Control & Prevention, Qiongzhong, Hainan, PR China
[j]Tunchang County Center for Disease Control & Prevention, Tunchang, Yunnan, PR China
[k]Ledong County Center for Disease Control & Prevention, Ledong, Hainan, PR China
[l]Changjiang County Center for Disease Control & Prevention, Changjiang, Hainan, PR China
[m]Baisha County Center for Disease Control & Prevention, Baisha, Hainan, PR China
*Corresponding authors: e-mail address: wangguangze63@126.com; ybdoctor@163.com; jkban702@163.com

Contents

1. Introduction 70
2. Background 72
   2.1 Programme for malaria control and elimination in Hainan 72
   2.2 Factors related to malaria transmission in Hainan 80
   2.3 Characteristics of forest goers that facilitate malaria transmission 85
3. The malaria surveillance and response system for forest goers in Hainan 88
   3.1 Recognition of forest goers as a high-risk population for malaria infection 88
   3.2 Outbreaks and sporadic cases in the control stage: Two retrospective case studies 88
   3.3 Transmission patterns and interventions in the elimination stage: A retrospective study on outbreaks in forest goers 95
   3.4 Imported cases and surveillance in the elimination stage: 2011–20 103

Advances in Parasitology, Volume 116
ISSN 0065-308X
https://doi.org/10.1016/bs.apar.2022.01.001

4. Ongoing challenges and responses in forest goers after malaria elimination in Hainan Province 108
4.1 Challenges in forest goers after malaria elimination in Hainan Province 108
4.2 Response in forest goers to malaria elimination in Hainan Province 109
Acknowledgements 109
References 110

Abstract

Hainan Province is in a tropical area of China and previously experienced serious *P. falciparum* and *P. vivax* malaria epidemics. After nearly 70 consecutive years of malaria prevention and control, malaria in Hainan has gradually been eliminated. To achieve the elimination of malaria, Hainan enacted six stages: investigative research and pilot prevention and control, large-scale antimalaria measures, adjustment of strategies for prevention and control, joint prevention and control measures, global funding of routine malaria control, and malaria elimination. Different strategies for malaria control were adopted at different stages. Malaria was most prevalent in the mountainous areas of central and southern Hainan, which contain a high-risk population (the forest goers) and two highly effective malaria vectors (*An. dirus* and *An. minimus*). Forest goers have been a high-risk population for malaria in Hainan since their identification in the 1990s. This paper summarizes malaria monitoring in forest goers and the response of forest goers to malaria control and elimination, distilling specific malaria control and elimination measures via case studies in Hainan Province. Two case studies in the malaria control stage demonstrated different measures for outbreaks and sporadic cases in forest goers. In view of the malaria outbreak in Sanya during the elimination stage, three-layered strategies (TLSs) were implemented to control outbreaks and improve control measures. Moreover, this paper also illustrates specific management measures to prevent malaria retransmission from sporadic imported malaria cases during the elimination phase. Hainan finally eliminated malaria in 2020. However, the risk of malaria retransmission is still high due to the prevalence of effective malaria vectors in Hainan, and forest goers are still a high-risk population for malaria retransmission.

1. Introduction

Hainan Province, also called Qiongzhou, is located in the southernmost part of mainland China. Hainan Province includes Hainan Island and nearby isles, including the Xisha Islands, Nansha Islands and Zhongsha Islands. Currently, Hainan has 4 prefecture-level cities, 5 county-level cities, 4 counties, 6 autonomous counties, and 218 towns, with a permanent resident population of 9.3432 million as of 2019. The Han, Li, Miao and Hui ethnic groups are native, while other ethnic groups have moved to Hainan after the Liberation of China (Fig. 1).

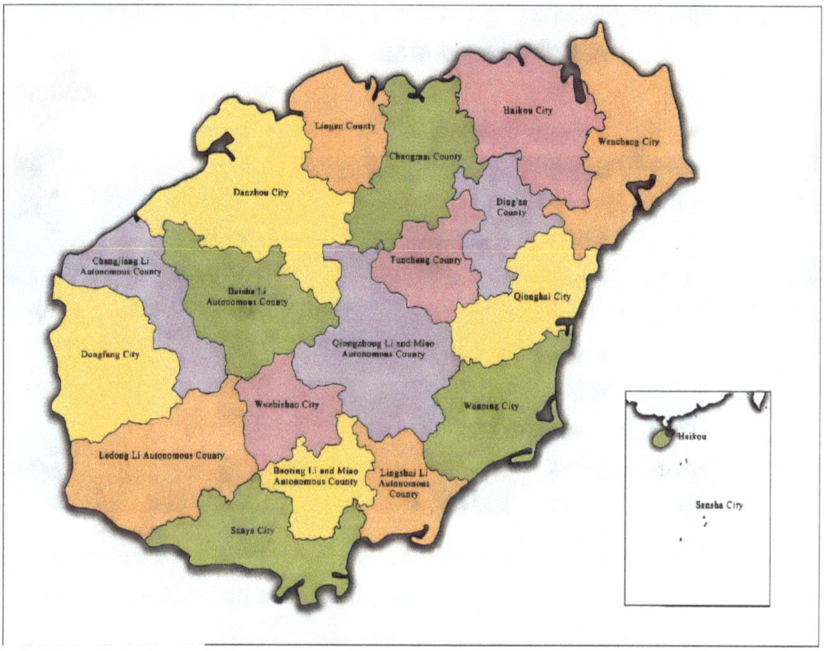

Fig. 1 A map of Hainan Province (The inset displays the included islands.)

Hainan Province previously had the highest incidence of malaria in China. Historically, the island was branded as 'the land of miasma' (Institute of Parasitic Diseases of Hainan Administrative Region, 1985; Wei et al., 2007). For example, a widespread poem describes the place: '*Ten thousand li they venture forth to Yazhou, but chances are slim that they will return from whence they came, for there lies death's door, where the living shudder to tread*'. Zhang Yuesong edited *Qiongzhou Government Records,* which states that in April of the 3rd year of the reign of Emperor Yongle (Ming Dynasty), reading '*Qiongzhou's mountains and rivers are perilous…few can survive the grasp of the vile miasma*'. Hainan was therefore seen as a hazardous place to visit.

Soon after the Liberation of China, malaria control specialists and epidemic control specialists conducted an in-depth survey of the rural areas of Hainan Island and recorded popular proverbs that reflected the epidemic situation at that time (Cai, 1993). For instance, '*Nanqiao and Lingshui are the two places from which visitors cannot return*' was widespread in the southeast, and '*The foot of Wuzhishan Mountain is a dismal place to live; there, ghosts outnumber the living, natural and man-made disasters wreak havoc and claim lives, until the blood and tears of the Miao and Li people flow like rivers*' was a popular saying among the ethnic groups of Miao and Li around Wuzhishan Mountain.

Starting in 1951, the Hainan provincial government emphasized malaria prevention and control and widely promoted malaria control and elimination measures. The province achieved a national certification of malaria elimination in 2019, and an independent WHO advisory team of experts certified malaria elimination in the field in 2021 (Ma, 2021). This achievement is due to the many studies on malaria prevention and control that were conducted over the years, including studies on the species distribution and dynamics of malaria cases and vectors. Importantly, forest goers were found to be more susceptible to malaria infection in Hainan (Lin et al., 1993), *Anopheles dirus* was found to the main vector of malaria transmission in the mountain forest area in Hainan Province (Chen et al., 2007) and insecticide-treated mosquito nets were invented and applied to prevent and control malaria in areas where *An. dirus* was prevalent (Si et al., 1993). Malaria infection among forest goers was also reported in the Greater Mekong subregion (Edwards et al., 2015; Hewitt, 2019).

Forest goers are defined as individuals, including local residents and migrants, who spend the night in the mountains for logging (Lin et al., 1994), planting (Si et al., 1994), gathering, etc., for profit or for subsistence (Wu et al., 1995). Forest goers were not only the main population infected with malaria during the malaria control stage in Hainan but also the main infected population during the malaria elimination stage (Wang, 2019). Therefore, this paper reviews the success of malaria control and elimination in forest goers through surveys and responses and identifies future risks and challenges.

2. Background

2.1 Programme for malaria control and elimination in Hainan

Starting in 1951, the Hainan government embarked on a half-century-long campaign of malaria prevention and control. The history of malaria prevention and control in Hainan can be divided into six stages: baseline surveys and key pilot programmes of malaria prevention and control (1951–57), large-scale antimalarial activity (1958–66), adjustment of strategies and improvements in management of malaria prevention and control (1967–91), joint prevention and control combined with pilot programmes (1992–2002), malaria control that combined the Global Fund with routine work (2003–10), and malaria elimination (2011–20) (Fig. 2).

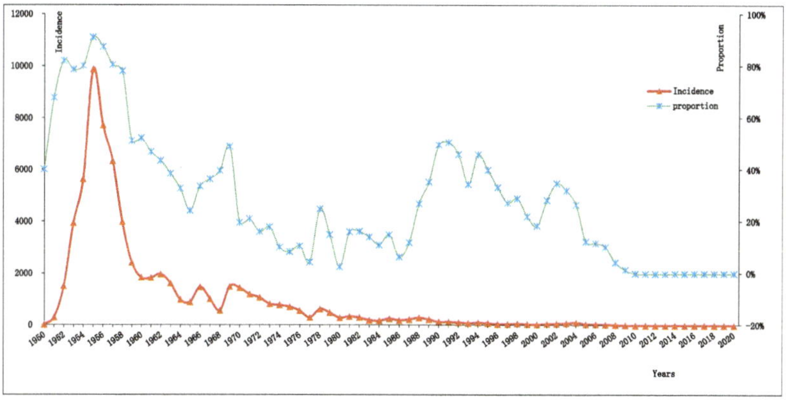

Fig. 2 Changes in the incidence of malaria and the proportion of malaria cases out of the total reported infectious disease cases from 1950 to 2020 in Hainan Province.

The prevalence of malaria, key prevention and control measures, and results and the achievements from each stage are summarized below.

2.1.1 Malaria baseline survey and key pilot programmes of malaria prevention and control (1951–57)

Since 1953, malaria investigations and pilot studies of prevention and control have been successively conducted by the Hainan Malaria Research Station of the Chinese Academy of Medical Sciences and by the Lei Qiong Malaria Prevention and Control stations in Xinglong, Lianchang, Nanfeng, Nanqiao, Liwan, Yacha and Maoyang (Hainan Island Committee Leading Office of Disease Eradication, 1962; He, 1965). In 1957, several professional teams were sent to carry out malaria investigations and research at a larger scale in Haikou, Qiongshan, Wenchang, Qiongdong, Lehui, Tunchang, Ding 'an, Chengmai, and Lingao as well as greater areas (Fig. 3). They found that the prevalence of the malaria parasite in residents was more than 50% in mountainous areas, approximately 30% in hilly areas, and less than 10% in plain areas. *P. falciparum* accounted for 52.6% of infections, *P. vivax* accounted for 24.2%, *P. malariae* accounted for 2.0%, and mixed infections accounted for 21.2%. In 1956, a case infected with *P. ovale* was found in Danzhou. In total, 37 species of anopheles mosquitoes were found in Hainan (Wei et al., 2007).

2.1.2 Large-scale antimalarial activity throughout the island (1958–66)

In 1958, a comprehensive antimalarial strategy was implemented in Hainan, with Lingshui and Baoting as the pilot counties (Baoting and Lingshui

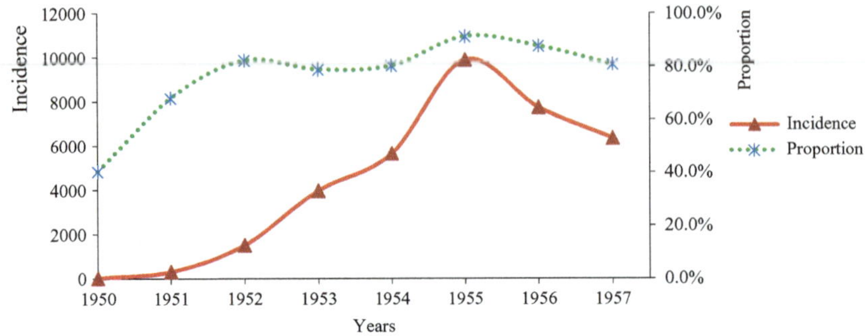

Fig. 3 Changes in the incidence of malaria and the proportion of malaria cases out of the total reported infectious disease cases in Hainan Province (1951–57).

Sanitary and Epidemic Control Station and Hainan Island Institute of Tropical Disease Control, 1962; Gao, 2009). According to the requirements of the 'Agricultural Development Program', an anti-malaria conference was held in Qiongzhong County in 1959, and antimalarial activities were subsequently deployed across the island (Institute of Parasitic Diseases of Hainan Administrative Region, 1985). Under the unified leadership of the district disease control office, offices were established in cities, counties, and towns to provide full-time malaria control staff, funds and equipment for antimalarial activities, and training courses for antimalarial personnel at the grassroots level. During the antimalarial campaign, the first secretary of each county led the antimalarial work, organized the antimalarial teams, and actively mobilized the public to implement insecticide residue spray(IRS) to kill *An. minimus* and to carry out mass drug administration (MDA) (Liu, 1957, 1960; Wu, 1960). After years of comprehensive antimalarial efforts, the annual incidence of malaria in Hainan decreased 78.52%, from 678.09 cases per ten thousand individuals in 1957 to 145.68 per ten thousand in 1966. The malaria mortality rate declined 68.97%, from 1.99 deaths per ten thousand cases in 1957 to 0.48 per ten thousand in 1966 (Fig. 4).

2.1.3 Adjustment of strategies and classifications to facilitate management of malaria prevention and control (1967–91)

Malaria stratification and corresponding antimalarial measures were updated according to malaria incidence, and the distribution and species of malaria vectors were recorded in four different zone (Cai, 1993; Cai et al., 1990a). Chloroquine plus primaquine was the main MDA drug combination, and DDT was the preferred insecticide for IRS. In Type I zones, where *An. dirus* and *An. minimus* were found year-round, the annual malaria

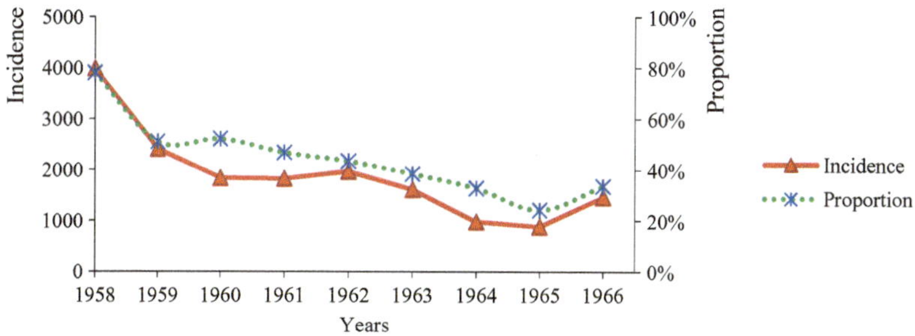

Fig. 4 Changes in the incidence of malaria and the proportion of malaria cases out of the total reported infectious disease cases throughout the island (1958–66).

incidence was 5–10%, and the parasitaemia rate was over 5%. In these zones, IRS and MDA were the primary strategies; IRS was implemented in spring and autumn each year and MDA was provided in the spring, summer and autumn each year. In Type II zones, where *An. minimus* was the main vector and *An. dirus* was occasionally found, the incidence of malaria was 1–5%, and the parasitaemia rate was 1–3%. In these zones, IRS and MDA were also the main strategies; IRS was implemented once a year in the spring, and MDA was administered in the spring and autumn each year. In Type III zones, where no *An. minimus* or *An. dirus* were found, both the incidence of malaria and the parasitaemia rate were less than 1%. In these zones, IRS was either implemented once a year or not at all, and MDA was administered only in high-risk villages. In Type IV zones, where no indigenous cases were found, only those who had a history of malaria or those who had parasites were treated with antimalaria drugs. However, chloroquine-resistant *P. falciparum* strains, which were discovered in 1974 (Cai et al., 1984), managed to spread to 11 counties, and malaria outbreaks occurred in some areas.

In the face of these chloroquine-resistant *P. falciparum* strains, four new malaria-endemic zones, using the village as a unit, were established in 1979 according to the prevalence of malaria and the distribution of vectors. Chloroquine plus primaquine was still the main MDA drug combination, and DDT plus DDV or fenitrothion were the preferred insecticides for IRS. In Type I zones, malaria outbreaks in mountainous villages were controlled, and IRS and MDA were implemented twice in the spring and autumn each year; the annual incidence of malaria was expected to decrease by more than 30%. In Type II zones, sporadic cases surrounding hilly villages were reduced, IRS was implemented once or twice a year, and MDA was carried out in villages with high incidence. In Type III zones, attention was

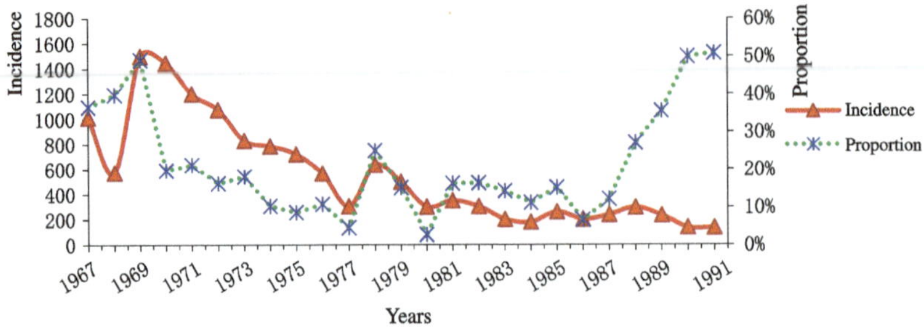

Fig. 5 Changes in the incidence of malaria and the proportion of malaria cases out of the total reported infectious disease cases throughout the island (1967–91).

focused on managing the migrant population and treating malaria patients, including radical treatments. In Type IV zones, effective surveillance and response to imported malaria outbreaks were maintained. During this time (1967–91), the incidence of malaria declined 87.80%, from 111.60 cases per ten thousand individuals in 1967 to 13.61 per ten thousand in 1991, and the mortality rate declined from 0.39 deaths per million (15 cases) in 1967 to 0.03 per million (2 cases) in 1991 (Fig. 5).

2.1.4 Joint prevention and control strategies combined with pilot programmes (1992–2002)

From 1992 to 2002, Hainan continued to enact comprehensive measures to control malaria, including seasonal IRS, case treatment and management, and the protection of susceptible populations. Every spring and autumn, malaria campaigns were carried out among high-risk populations, which included implementation of MDA and IRS and the administration of ITNs. In particular, the introduction of ITNs treated with deltamethrin and naphthoquinone phosphate (Cai et al., 1990a,b; Si et al., 1993; Wu et al., 2001) in susceptible populations substantially reduced malaria cases, as did timely intervention in malaria epidemic foci and outbreaks. Teams for malaria prevention and control were developed in prefectural or county CDCs, township hospitals, and rural health clinics in villages; these teams improved malaria surveillance and response at all levels. Moreover, 10 townships in four counties (Wanning, Qiongzhong, Baoting and Ledong), including 73,100 people, jointly combated malaria starting in 1984 and expanded their coverage to include over 1.6 million people in 14 cities or counties by 1992. In 1992, a malaria prevention network targeting migrant populations was established in Guangdong, Guangxi and Hainan (Wang et al., 2013). Additionally, in 1991, 10 townships in 10 counties or cities, including Wanning, Lingshui and Sanya, with the highest incidence of malaria were selected for pilot studies on malaria prevention and control to facilitate antimalarial research (Cai and Cai, 1996; Si et al., 1998). Decreases in the incidence of malaria in these pilot areas directly resulted in a decline in malaria incidence in Hainan. In particular, forest goers, who overnight in the mountains, were identified as a high-risk population. However, during this period, many people moved to mountainous areas in the central and southern parts of the province where *P. falciparum* was prevalent (Cai and Cai, 1998), resulting in a rise in malaria morbidity and mortality in some years (Wu et al., 1998). However, the overall incidence of malaria during this period declined by 87.8%, from 11.46 cases per 10,000 individuals in 1992 to 692 per 10,000 in 2002, and the number of deaths fell from 4 in 1992 to 1 in 2002 (Fig. 6).

2.1.5 Combination of the Global Fund's malaria programme with routine malaria control work (2003–10)

Round 1 of the Global Fund's malaria projects (GF-1) started in 10 Hainan counties and cities with high malaria prevalence in 2003, lasting until 2008 (Ma, 2010). The number of *P. falciparum* malaria cases in Hainan dropped from 857 in 2003 to 30 in 2008 and this period also created conditions that favoured the elimination of *P. falciparum*. Round 5 of the Global Fund's malaria projects (GF-5) started in 16 Hainan cities and counties in 2006; the number of malaria cases, including *P. falciparum* and *P. vivax,* decreased from 3852 in 2006 to 78 in 2010, progressing towards the goal of malaria elimination (Lin and Weng, 2013). In 2010, no indigenous cases of *P. falciparum* malaria were reported (Sun et al., 2015). The Global Fund of National Strategic Application (NSA) for malaria projects started in

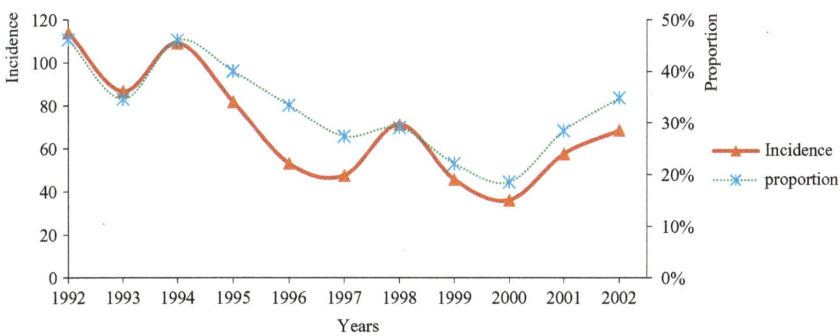

Fig. 6 Changes in the incidence of malaria and the proportion of malaria cases out of the total reported infectious disease cases (1992–2002).

2010 and covered 18 cities and counties in Hainan Province (Xu, 2014); thus, the malaria epidemic in the project area was significantly contained. By 2012, no indigenous cases of malaria were reported in Hainan Province. The strategies for malaria prevention and control were as follows. First, the prevalence and spread of *P. falciparum* malaria in high-transmission areas was reduced by focusing on the migrant population, mountain residents and forest goers. Second, outbreak control and transmission were reduced by timely identification of the source of infection, outbreak control and radical treatment in unstable epidemic areas. Third, imported malaria or residual indigenous cases were prevented from spreading by focusing on timely detection of sources of infection followed by standard antimalarial treatment in areas where the epidemic was effectively contained, such as Haikou City in Lingao County (Zeng, 2015). Pilot projects, joint prevention and control programmes, and seasonal antimalarial activities were carried out. Additionally, the use of ITNs with deltamethrin and insecticide long-lasting nets (ILLNs) was promoted, along with rapid diagnostic tests and artemisinin-based combination treatments.

During this period, the incidence of malaria decreased 98.85%, from 7.84 cases per 10,000 individuals in 2003 to 0.09 per 10,000 in 2010, and the number of deaths decreased from 1 in 2003 to 0 in 2010, laying a solid foundation for the elimination of malaria in Hainan Province. Compared to the incidence of malaria in 2003, the number of malaria cases in 2004 increased by 32.22% due to the improvement in malaria detection and reductions in underreporting after the implementation of those projects; these numbers soon decreased (Fig. 7).

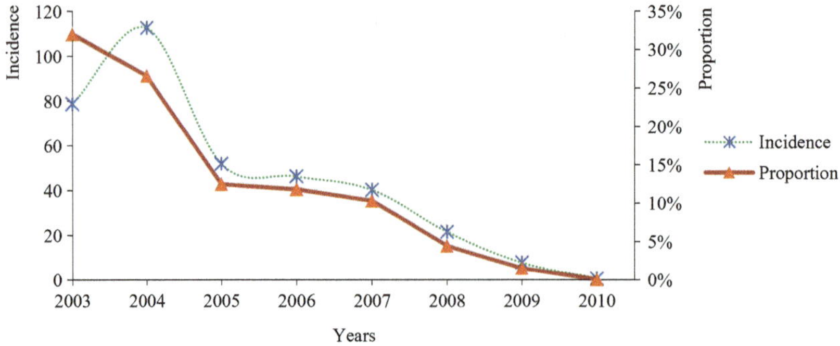

Fig. 7 Changes in the incidence of malaria and the proportion of malaria cases out of the total reported infectious disease cases throughout the island (2003–10).

2.1.6 Achievement of malaria elimination (2011–20)

The malaria elimination campaign in Hainan started in October 2010 with the release of the China Malaria Elimination Action Plan (Xia et al., 2014). At that time, out of 18 cities and counties in Hainan, 10 were classified as Type I zones (Sanya City, LingShui County, Wuzhishan City, Ledong County, Wanning City, Dongfang City, BaoTing County, Qiaongzhong County, Changjiang County and Baisha County) and 8 were classified as Type II zones (Haikou City, Wenchang City, Qianghai City, Ding'an County, Dunchang County, Chengmai County, Lingao County and Danzhou City). Comprehensive prevention and control strategies focusing on the control of infectious sources were carried out in all Type I and II cities and counties, supplemented by vector control and increased protection of susceptible populations (Wang, 2019).

From 2011 to 2020, 99 malaria cases were reported in Hainan Province, including 1 death, 11 indigenous malaria cases, and 88 imported malaria cases. The majority of indigenous malaria cases (72.73%; 8/11) were in Sanya, while other cities and counties accounted for 27.27% (3/11). Of the 88 imported malaria cases, 69 were from Mozambique or other African countries, and 19 were from Cambodia or other southeast Asian countries. In 2009 and 2012 (Sun et al., 2016), *P. falciparum* and *P. vivax* were successively eliminated in Hainan (Zhang et al., 2016). In 2015, local transmission of *P. malariae* was successfully blocked. Since 2016, no indigenous malaria cases have been reported (Wang, 2019). All cities and counties passed the provincial malaria elimination assessment in 2018 (Fig. 8).

Starting in 2012, Hainan implemented the 1-3-7 approach for malaria elimination, namely, reporting malaria cases within 24h (1 day), conducting case reviews and epidemic investigations within 3 days, and investigating

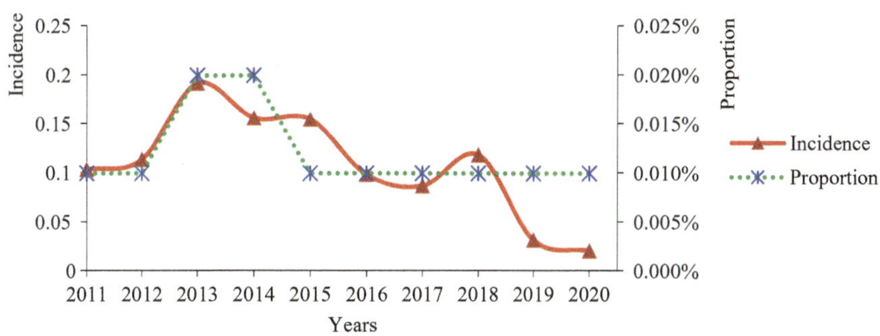

Fig. 8 Changes in the incidence of malaria and the proportion of malaria cases out of the total reported infectious disease cases (2011–20).

Table 1 Implementation of the 1-3-7 approach in Hainan Province from 2011 to 2020.

Year	Reported cases	Interval between onset of fever and diagnosis (days)	Interval between diagnosis and report (<24h)	Interval between epidemic investigation and report (<3 days)	Interval between the disposal of the foci and report (<7 days)
2011[a]	9[a]	8.3	24.00	2.0	2.0
2012[b]	13	5.9	11.69	1.0	24.6
2013	16	11.2	11.14	0.9	2.4
2014	13	5.1	10.92	0.9	2.5
2015[a]	15[a]	3.3	10.00	0.8	2.8
2016	8	2.6	8.37	0.7	1.2
2017	8	7.9	15.58	1.3	2.5
2018	11	3.4	10.82	0.9	1.5
2019	3	2.7	13.00	1.1	1.8
2020	3	0.8	19.67	1.6	3.2
Average	10	5.8	12.21	1.0	5.7

[a]Indigenous malaria was found in this year.
[b]The '1-3-7' approach, which was launched in 2012, involves reporting cases within 1 day, investigating cases within 3 days, and disposal of the foci within 7 days.

and treating foci within 7 days. The rate of malaria reporting within 24 h was 98.9%, the epidemiological investigation completion rate within 3 days was 100%, and the epidemic site investigation and treatment rate within 7 days was 100% (Table 1).

To date, malaria control and elimination has been carried out for nearly 70 years; Hainan achieved a national certification of malaria elimination in 2019 and a WHO field certification of malaria elimination in 2021 (Ma, 2021). Thus, Hainan has shifted from the 'Land of Miasma' to today's 'Island of Health' (Fig. 9).

2.2 Factors related to malaria transmission in Hainan

2.2.1 Natural factors

Hainan Province has a tropical monsoon climate and boasts abundant rainfall, with an average annual precipitation of 1639 mm. Hainan Island has a lower peripheral altitude and a higher centre, featuring Wuzhi Mountain

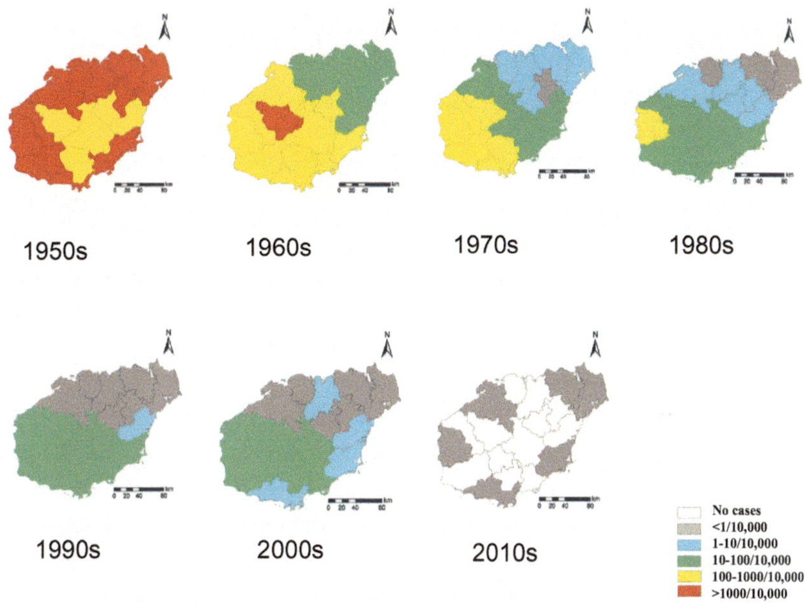

Fig. 9 Malaria incidence (number of cases per 10,000 individuals) in Hainan Province from 1950 to 2020.

and Yingge Mountain; mountains ranging from 500 to 800 m and plains circle the centre. These natural environmental and climatic conditions not only support high forest coverage and rich growth in the mountain forests of Hainan but also provide a natural environment for the reproduction of malaria vectors.

2.2.2 Vector species characteristics

Historically, a total of 37 species of anopheles mosquitoes have been identified in Hainan, of which 6 species were regarded as primary or secondary vectors for malaria transmission in the 1950s, including *An. minimus*, *An. dirus*, *An. fluviatilis*, *An. jeyporiensis candidiensis*, *An. philippinensis*, and *An. sinensis* (Pan, 2003). Positive infection with plasmodium sporozoites was identified in the salivary glands of wild individuals of *An. minumus*, *An. dirus*, *An. rivieri*, *An. helioides*, *An. phillipidae* and *An. sinensis* captured at survey sites (Hainan Island District Party Committee Leading Group Office of Disease Eradication, 1962; Institute of Parasitic Diseases of Hainan Administrative Region, 1985; Sheng, 1957; Zhou, 1957). Of these species, *An. minumus* and *An. dirus* feed on human blood, *An. minimus* prefers urban areas and is distributed throughout towns in Hainan, and *An. dirus* prefers rural areas and is only found in forested areas (Institute of Parasitic Diseases of Hainan Administrative Region, 1985). *An. minumus* has a large population in Hainan, and sporozoites were observed in their salivary glands in all months. This species was the main malaria vector in Hainan. In addition, a positive rate of 3.5% in *An. minumus* and 4.3% in *An. dirus* were found in the wild in Xinglong, Nanqiao, Lianchang, Nanfeng, Baisha and other places in 1955.

An. minimus and *An. dirus* were the primary malaria vectors in Hainan and were mainly found in the forests in the southern and central parts of the province (Fig. 10).

An. minimus was identified as the main vector of malaria in the 1950s; it was the dominant mosquito species in urban areas and preferred human blood (Institute of Parasitic Diseases of Hainan Administrative Region, 1985). It was found in 18 counties or cities across the island, and was sensitive to DDT (He, 1956). *An. minimus* was essentially contained island-wide after several years of IRS, from 1963 to 1965 (He et al., 1964). After the 1970s, its distribution gradually increased again, mainly in Danzhou City, Baisha County, Changjiang County, and Dongfang City. In the 1980s, *An. minimus* gradually spread to the central and eastern parts of the island. In the 1990s, it was found in all cities and counties across the island. From 2000 to 2010, *An. minimus* distribution was shrink to 10 cities and counties, including Wuzhishan City, Chengmai County, Lingshui County, Wanning City, Baoting County, Ledong County, Dongfang City, Baisha County, Tunchang County and Changjiang County. *An. minimus* distribution was further reduced to 7 cities and counties from 2011 to 2020, including

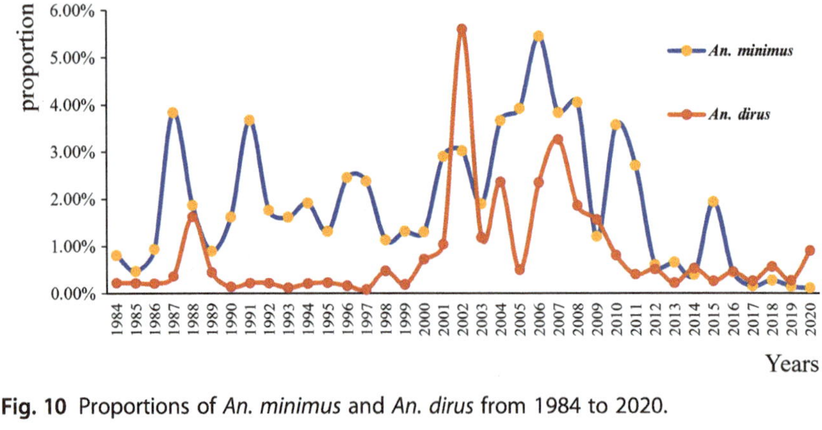

Fig. 10 Proportions of *An. minimus* and *An. dirus* from 1984 to 2020.

Wuzhishan City, Qiongzhong County, Baoting County, Dongfang City, Baisha County, Tunchang County and Changjiang County. Peak levels of *An. minimus* occur from April to June. In some areas, a small peak occurs in September and October due to local rainfall (Li, 1997). *An. minimus* is active all night, and its activity peak is at approximately midnight. Moreover, the blood-sucking activity of *An. minimus* increases sharply after 22:00 and peaks at 23:00–00:00. *An. minimus* behaviour in the 1990s differed from that in the 1950s in terms of blood-sucking and roosting; although they fed on cattle blood, they could still cause local malaria transmission or outbreaks (Lin et al., 2009). IRS with DDT and INTs with deltamethrin effectively controlled the population of *An. minimus* (Li, 1997) (Fig. 11).

Compared with *An. minimus*, *An. dirus* was mainly found in mountainous areas and nearby hilly areas. In the 1950s, *An. dirus* was found in the mountainous areas of all 15 counties or cities except Haikou, Wenchang and coastal areas (Institute of Parasitic Diseases of Hainan Administrative Region, 1985). After *An. minimus* was effectively contained in 1962, *An. dirus* became the main vector of malaria transmission in mountainous or hilly forested areas. From 1963 to 1970, it was mainly found in mountainous and hilly areas. Since the 1970s, the distribution of *An. dirus* has shrunk and the population of *An. dirus* has decreased (Wu et al., 1998). From 1980 to 1989,

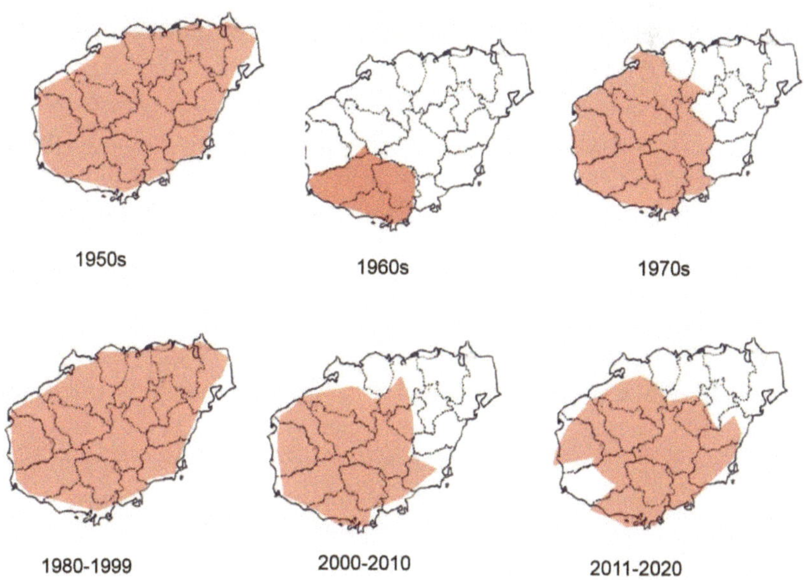

Fig. 11 Distributions of *An. minimus* on Hainan Island during the past 70 years.

An. dirus was found in nine counties or cities, including Wuzhishan City, Qiongzhong County, Chengmai County, Lingshui County, Wanning City, Baoting County, Ledong County, Baisha County and Changjiang County. The distribution of *An. dirus* was similar to that in the 1980s from 1990 to 1999 (Hainan Institute of Tropical Disease Control, 2000). In 2000 to 2010, *An. dirus* was mainly found in eight cities or counties, including Wuzhishan City, Qiongzhong County, Ledong County, Wanning City, Baoting County, Dongfang City, Baisha County and Changjiang County. In 2011 to 2020, the distribution of *An. dirus* was reduced and it was mainly found in five counties or cities, including Wuzhishan City, Qiongzhong County, Baoting County, Baisha County and Changjiang County.

In 1982, the peak activity of *An. dirus* was from May to October (Institute of Parasitic Diseases of Hainan Administrative Region, 1985). *An. dirus* could be captured in all months, but its peak activity was in July (Lin et al., 2000). *An. dirus* appears in Wuzhishan City every month, with peak activity from March to July. However, from 2004 to 2014, *An. dirus* appeared at the monitoring site of Beiwan village, Qiongzhong from February to November, and its peak activity was in August.

The biting and bloodsucking activities of *An. dirus* are concentrated around midnight. In the 1980s, its earliest time of appearance in the village was 19:30, its peak activity was 22:00–01:00, and its activity stopped at 5:00, but biting activity was also found in the dense forest during the daytime. In 2003, similarly, the peak activity of *An. dirus* at night lasted from 21:00 to 4:00 a.m., and the peak of biting activity was 22:00–2:00 p.m.

In addition, *An. dirus* in Hainan Province belongs to species A (Xu and Qu, 1997). *An. dirus* is sensitive to the DDT, and its flight radius is approximately 1.5 km (Li et al., 1990; Su et al., 1985). Because *An. dirus* is difficult to control, it is the primary cause of infection in forest goers (Cai, 1993) (Fig. 12) (Table 2).

2.2.3 Malaria species characteristics

Historically, *P. vivax*, *P. falciparum*, *P. malariae* and *P. ovale* were found in Hainan. In general, *P. falciparum* and *P. vivax* were common indigenous malaria cases, while *P. malariae* was scattered and *P. ovale* was rare. Indigenous malaria was mainly distributed in central and southern cities and counties, while the prevalence was low in cities and counties on the coastal plain. *P. falciparum* was mainly distributed in 10 cities and counties where ethnic minorities lived, and *P. vivax* was distributed throughout the island prior to 2012.

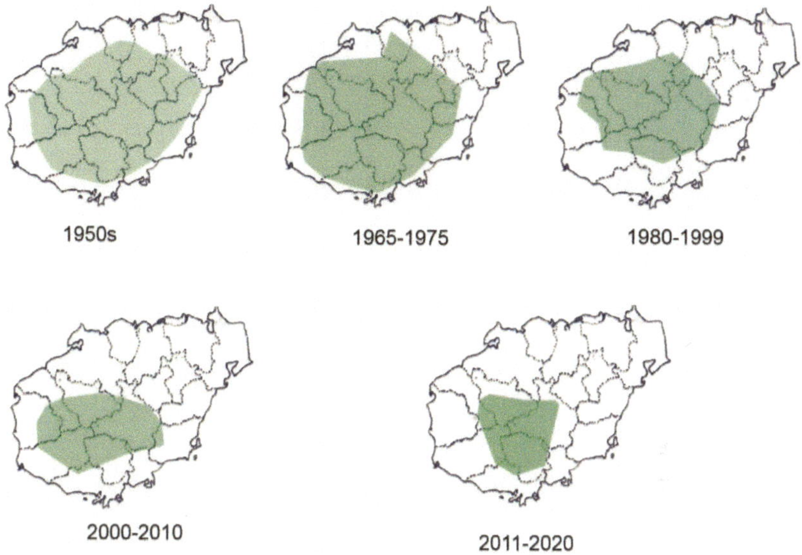

Fig. 12 Distributions of *An. dirus* in Hainan Island during the past 70 years.

2.3 Characteristics of forest goers that facilitate malaria transmission

Forest goers, who overnight in the mountains (Tang et al., 1995), are susceptible to malaria infection, particularly *P. falciparum* infection, and become the main source of malaria infection in mountainous areas of central Hainan (Fig. 13). This 'mountain infection' carried by forest goers in Hainan was more serious than village infection (Lin et al., 1993; Wang, 1997, Wang et al., 1998). In 1991, 60.8% (5306/8715) of malaria cases were forest goers in Hainan, a significant increase from 53.2% in 1990 (Si et al., 1992). Moreover, the infection rate among forest goers in Wanning was six times that of the population of villagers (Lin et al., 1993). Additionally, the relative risk (RR) of malaria was 6.5 times higher for people who visit to the forest frequently and 4.2 times higher for people who had previously visited the forest (Wu et al., 1998). The reasons for increased susceptibility in forest goers are described below.

2.3.1 Living in housing that is easy for mosquitoes to enter

Forest goers live in scattered houses or variations on simple shanties, mostly with bamboo walls (or no walls) and grass roofs (Lin et al., 1993); This population overnights in shanties (13.87%), huts (55.16%) or outdoors (28.06%)

Table 2 Comparison of the distribution and behaviours of *An. dirus* and *An. minimus.*

Vector species	Period and place	Activity		Host species	Place of capture	Insecticide used in IRS
		Over months	Over the day			
An. minimus	1950s: 18 counties or cities			Prefers human blood	Human housing	DDT
	1960s: virtually contained					
	1970s: distribution increased					
	1980s: in central and eastern parts of the island					
	1990s: across the island	April to June, small peak in September and October		Human and cattle blood	Cattle housing	DDT and deltamethrin
	2000s: 10 cities and counties		Midnight			
	2010s: 10 cities and counties					
An. dirus	1950s: all 15 counties or cities except Haikou, Wenchang and coastal areas.				Wild-dwelling	
	1960s: mountainous and hilly areas					
	1970s: distribution shrunk and population decreased					
	1980s: nine counties or cities	May to October	Peak: 22:00–01:00, activity stopped by 5:00			
	1990s: similar to that in the 1980s	All months, peak activity in July	Earliest appearance at 19:30, peak activity from 22:00 to 23:00; biting activity also found during the day			DDT
	2000s: eight cities or counties	March to July	21:00 to 4:00 a.m., peak biting at 22:00–2:00 p.m.			
	2010s: five counties or cities					

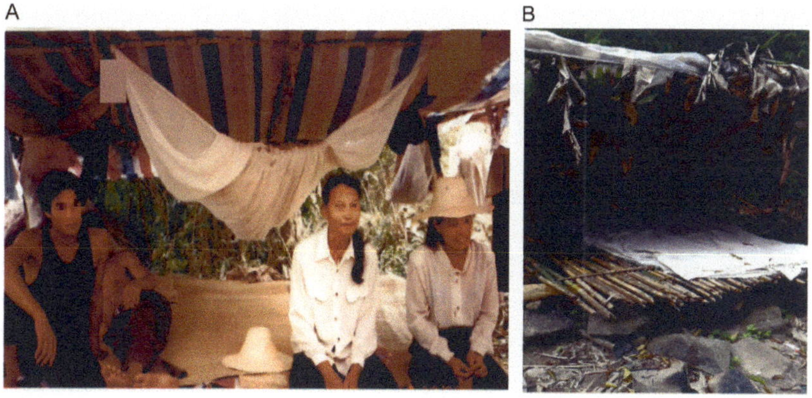

Fig. 13 Forest goer housing. (A) Photo from Dongfang in 2000; (B) Photo from Sanya in 2015.

when they were in the forest (He et al., 2012). This housing is close to mosquito breeding grounds, and no cattle or other livestock are present (Wang et al., 2002), resulting in a significant increase in human mosquito bites (Wu et al., 1995). The biting rate of *An. dirus* was 27.2 times higher in shanty areas (13.28 per person/night) than in villages (0.47 per person/night) in Heping Town in Qiongzhong County (Lin et al., 2000).

2.3.2 Lack of mosquito nets or lower rates of mosquito net use

Most forest goers did not use mosquito nets, or the mosquito net utilization rate in forest goers was lower (Lin et al., 2005). In other words, the use of mosquito nets is one of the main factors affecting the control of malaria and increasing both the implementation of mosquito nets and their use can greatly reduce the forest goer exposure and the vector energy of mosquitoes in forest goers (Chen et al., 1995; He et al., 2012). Moreover, increasing both the implementation of mosquito nets and their use can greatly reduce the forest goer exposure and the vector energy of mosquitoes in forest goers, along with the use of deltamethrin in *An. dirus*- and *An. minimus*-dominated areas (Lin and Li, 1999).

2.3.3 Lack of malaria prevention knowledge

A lack of knowledge about malaria prevention was the main risk factor for malaria infection (Chen et al., 1995), and health education was conducted to influence the behaviour of high-risk populations through increased understanding (Lin et al., 2001). Malaria health education was carried out, and the rate of correct answers from residents on malaria knowledge tests increased from 61.3% to 89.7% after health education. The rate of mosquito net use increased from 28.6% to 72.6%, and the malaria index in pilot townships dropped to a low level. Moreover, the usage of rate in preventive medicine use among forest goers was increased (Lin et al., 2005).

2.3.4 Weakness of treatment adherence

Weakness in malaria treatment compliance was found in forest goers. Only 16.1% of patients took primaquine for the prescription-specific 4 days (Wu et al., 1998). Moreover, the number of people receiving the standard malaria treatment was only 0.2% (2 cases), but the number of people receiving treatments accounted for 96.3% (1219 cases) (Lin et al., 2005). Improving compliance with malaria treatment and standardizing malaria treatment can reduce the source of infection (Chen et al., 1999).

3. The malaria surveillance and response system for forest goers in Hainan

3.1 Recognition of forest goers as a high-risk population for malaria infection

The malaria incidence and mortality rate in Hainan decreased over time, accompanied by a shrinkage in the distribution of *An. minimus* from 18 cities and counties in 1958 to 7 cities and counties before 1978. However, malaria infection is still a serious issue in mountainous areas; *An. dirus* is the main malaria vector in these areas and is difficult to reduce by IRS. During 1980s, a large number of nonlocal workers entered Hainan for new projects constructing or crop planting, and the malaria incidence rose significantly.

Since 1991, 10 malaria control pilots in 10 counties, including Wanning, Lingshui and Sanya, have been set up in townships with high malaria incidence to understand the causes of the rising malaria incidence. In these pilots, the species of malaria parasite were recorded for each malaria case, and the source of infection was also investigated for foci disposal (Table 3).

Furthermore, forest goers were identified as the main victims of malaria infection, and their overnight behaviour may be the key factor of malaria infection (Table 4).

3.2 Outbreaks and sporadic cases in the control stage: Two retrospective case studies

During the malaria control stage, there were several outbreaks reported in high-epidemic areas (Duan et al., 1999; He et al., 1993; Si et al., 1995;

Table 3 Epidemiological surveillance data of malaria from 10 pilots between 1991 and 2011.

										Source of infection							
Year	Population	No. of report cases	API	NEBS	SPR	No. of *Pf*	*Pf*IR	No. of *Pv*	*Pv*IR	From villages	%	From mountains	%	From other counties	%	Unknown	%
1991[a]	59,887	1700	283.9	11,990	2.8%	713	119.1	985	164.5	599	35.2%	680	40.0%	51	3.0%	370	21.8%
1992	100,629	1452	144.3	18,482	1.4%	891	88.5	556	55.3	316	21.8%	1041	71.7%	14	1.0%	81	5.6%
1993	99,565	1049	105.4	17,953	1.1%	749	75.2	295	29.6	144	13.7%	531	50.6%	12	1.1%	61	5.8%
1994	101,060	1029	101.8	19,096	1.0%	743	73.5	284	28.1	124	12.1%	840	81.6%	19	1.8%	46	4.5%
1995	101,122	690	68.2	19,802	0.7%	510	50.4	178	17.6	65	9.4%	605	87.7%	2	0.3%	18	2.6%
1996	102,045	452	44.3	19,196	0.4%	349	34.2	103	10.1	30	6.6%	418	92.5%	1	0.2%	3	0.7%
1997	102,722	391	38.1	19,791	0.4%	266	25.9	121	11.8	39	10.0%	331	84.7%	7	1.8%	14	3.6%
1998	102,538	568	55.4	22,088	0.6%	424	41.4	143	13.9	65	11.4%	373	65.7%	115	20.2%	15	2.6%
1999	101,448	398	39.2	20,274	0.4%	307	30.3	91	9.0	33	8.3%	346	86.9%	7	1.8%	12	3.0%
2000	99,144	199	20.1	18,871	0.2%	145	14.6	54	5.4	19	9.5%	166	83.4%	6	3.0%	8	4.0%
2001	99,069	263	26.5	17,283	0.3%	175	17.7	87	8.8	13	4.9%	234	89.0%	14	5.3%	2	0.8%
2002	101,437	439	43.3	17,183	0.4%	314	31.0	125	12.3	18	4.1%	392	89.3%	25	5.7%	4	0.9%
2003	101,626	665	65.4	17,557	0.7%	535	52.6	130	12.8	35	5.3%	619	93.1%	7	1.1%	4	0.6%

Continued

Table 3 Epidemiological surveillance data of malaria from 10 pilots between 1991 and 2011.—cont'd

										Source of infection							
Year	Population	No. of report cases	API	NEBS	SPR	No. of *Pf*	*Pf*IR	No. of *Pv*	*Pv*IR	From villages	%	From mountains	%	From other counties	%	Unknown	%
2004	102,592	842	82.1	20,522	0.8%	612	59.7	230	22.4	23	2.7%	795	94.4%	15	1.8%	9	1.1%
2005	102,031	340	33.3	18,056	0.3%	293	28.7	47	4.6	15	4.4%	303	89.1%	0	0.0%	22	6.5%
2006	95,441	177	18.5	19,755	0.2%	165	17.3	12	1.3	24	13.6%	143	80.8%	9	5.1%	1	0.6%
2007	101,699	167	16.4	26,281	0.2%	161	15.8	6	0.6	13	7.8%	150	89.8%	0	0.0%	4	2.4%
2008	108,950	65	6.0	15,826	0.1%	64	5.9	1	0.1	2	3.1%	61	93.8%	0	0.0%	2	3.1%
2009	108,108	25	2.3	20,077	0.0%	25	2.3	0	0.0	1	4.0%	20	80.0%	0	0.0%	4	16.0%
2010	110,073	2	0.2	17,085	0.0%	2	0.2	0	0.0	0	0.0%	1	50.0%	0	0.0%	1	50.0%
2011	99,753	1	0.1	10,351	0.0%	1	0.1	0	0.0	0	0.0%	0	0.0%	1	100.0%	0	0.0%

[a]Does not include data from Sanya Gaofeng, Changjiang Qicha, or Dongfang Donghe.

NEBS: number of examinations by blood slides; API: annual parasite incidence; SPR: slide positive ratio; *Pf*IR: annual parasite incidence in *P. falciparum*; *Pv*IR: Number of *P. vivax* cases. Ten malaria control bases were established in Sanya Gaofeng, Lingshui Qunying, Changjiang Qicha, Wuzhishan Maoyang, Qiongzhong Heping, Wanning Nanqiao, Baoting Nanlin, Ledong Fubao, Baisha Qingsong, and Dongfang Donghe.

Table 4 Epidemiological surveillance data of malaria in reported cases in Hainan between 1991 and 2009.

				Source of infection							
Years	No. of RC	No. of ICRC	%	From villages	%	From mountains	%	From other counties or aboard	%	Unknown	%
1984	10,452	1106	10.6%	478	43.22%	443	40.05%	182	16.46%	3	0.27%
1985	15,501	1653	10.7%	603	36.48%	771	46.64%	279	16.88%	0	0.00%
1986	12,274	1058	8.6%	285	26.94%	304	28.73%	264	24.95%	5	0.47%
1987	14,426	2872	19.9%	694	24.16%	1769	61.59%	409	14.24%	0	0.00%
1990	9054	8712	96.2%	2688	30.85%	4632	53.17%	870	9.99%	522	5.99%
1991	9003	8711	96.8%	2127	24.42%	5306	60.91%	598	6.86%	680	7.81%
1992	7656	6863	89.6%	1291	18.81%	4795	69.87%	548	7.98%	229	3.34%
1993	6080	7139	117.4%	947	13.27%	4865	68.15%	202	2.83%	1125	15.76%
1994	7764	7423	95.6%	844	11.37%	4800	64.66%	204	2.75%	1575	21.22%
1995	5875	4875	83.0%	458	9.39%	3742	76.76%	117	2.40%	558	11.45%
1996	3906	3962	101.4%	219	5.53%	2694	68.00%	95	2.40%	954	24.08%
1997	3546	3014	85.0%	175	5.81%	2276	75.51%	86	2.85%	477	15.83%
1998	5379	3761	69.9%	233	6.20%	2677	71.18%	268	7.13%	583	15.50%
1999	3455	2338	67.7%	140	5.99%	1842	78.79%	55	2.35%	301	12.87%
2000	2734	3068	112.2%	164	5.35%	2510	81.81%	166	5.41%	228	7.43%

Continued

Table 4 Epidemiological surveillance data of malaria in reported cases in Hainan between 1991 and 2009.—cont'd

				Source of infection							
Years	**No. of RC**	**No. of ICRC**	**%**	**From villages**	**%**	**From mountains**	**%**	**From other counties or aboard**	**%**	**Unknown**	**%**
2001	4679	4676	99.9%	308	6.59%	3978	85.07%	144	3.08%	246	5.26%
2002	5509	4730	85.9%	348	7.36%	3594	75.98%	284	6.00%	504	10.66%
2003	6357	5552	87.3%	314	5.66%	4766	85.84%	154	2.77%	318	5.73%
2004	9193	9038	98.3%	164	1.81%	8328	92.14%	116	1.28%	430	4.76%
2005	4516	3788	83.9%	278	7.34%	3338	88.12%	62	1.64%	110	2.90%
2006[a]	3853	2135	55.4%	353	16.53%	1704	79.81%	12	0.56%	66	3.09%
2007	3387	2347	69.3%	384	16.36%	1902	81.04%	1	0.04%	60	2.56%
2008	1844	392	21.3%	48	12.24%	328	83.67%	0	0.00%	16	4.08%
2009	685	148	21.6%	5	3.38%	135	91.22%	2	1.35%	6	4.05%

[a]Clinically diagnosed cases were included in the report system since 2006. Until 2011, when the malaria elimination strategy was launched, every clinically diagnosed case was verified by a Reference Laboratory for Malaria Diagnosis.
RC: reported cases; ICRC: investigated cases of reported cases. Data from 1988 and 1989 are missing.

Zhou, 1980) but not in low-epidemic areas. Five outbreaks from 1984 to 1996 were transmitted by *An. minimus*, mainly due to the introduction of imported malaria cases (Lin et al., 2009): three occurred in coastal plain areas, and the other two occurred in hilly areas where indigenous malaria had not been detected for many years. Mainly, IRS and MDA were implemented to control the outbreaks. An outbreak of *P. falciparum* malaria among forest goers in Dongfang in 2000 is examined as Case Study I, and sporadic cases of *P. vivax* among forest goers in Baisha are examined as Case Study II.

Case Study I: Dongfang city, located in southwestern Hainan Province, had prevalent *P. falciparum* malaria. Jiangbian township, a remote township in Dongfang city, adjoins a large dam reservoir. In this township, there are the increased mountainous areas, dense tropical forest and mild climate, favour for the reproduction of *An. dirus* and *An. minimus*; The kinds of *P. falciparum* in this township were the most serious malaria in Dongfang (Wen et al., 1997). In particular, an outbreak occurred in a migrant population of forest goers in 2000 (Zhan, 2006; Zhu, 2002), when a forestry company recruited a large number of migrant workers from Hunan, Jiangxi, Anhui, Guizhou and other provinces to directly enter Jiangbian township to plant trees (and thus work as forest goers). In July, more than 20 of these migrant workers were infected with *P. falciparum* malaria, and 6 patients died after returning home to Wuyuan County, Jiangxi Province. Subsequently, 52 of these 78 forest goers came down with malaria, including 37 cases of *P. falciparum* malaria and 15 cases of *P. vivax* malaria (Fig. 14). An epidemiological survey of these migrant workers showed that they did not take preventive medicine and that they lived in unprotected housing that allowed easy access by mosquitos. Moreover, they overnighted without nets, and the vectors *An. minimus* and *An. dirus* were captured in their housing. *P. falciparum* malaria cases were treated with piperaquine plus primaquine, and *P. vivax* malaria cases were treated with chloroquine plus primaquine. During this outbreak, piperaquine was administered to every forest goer to prevent malaria, and the use of nets was encouraged. Since the implementation of these comprehensive measures, the number of malaria cases in Jiangbian decreased every month, from 52 cases in July to 5 in December. In this outbreak, the monitoring system had limited sensitivity, because that it was based on paper cards for reporting cases and only reports of surveillance data by monthly; Thus, malaria prevalence could be seriously underreported. Moreover, low levels of malaria diagnosis and treatment were found in remote township hospitals, such as Jiangbian, although some cases were admitted to local hospitals.

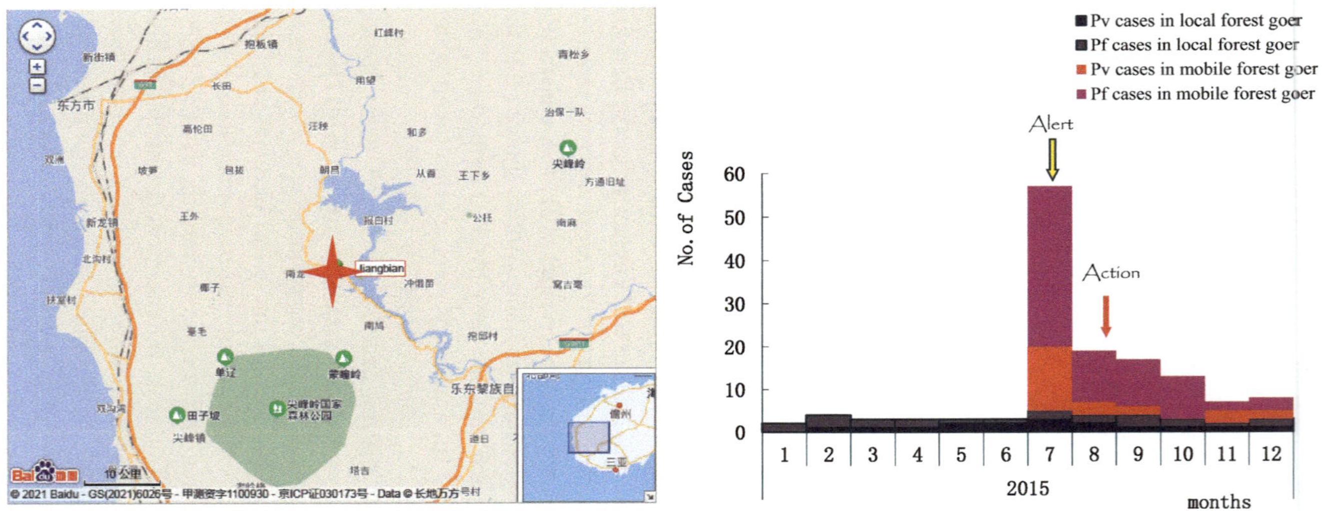

A

B

Fig. 14 The outbreak of *P. falciparum* among forest goers in Dongfang in 2000. (A) Location of Jiangban township in Dongfang, Hainan. (B) Surveillance, response and action in this outbreak.

Case Study II: Baisha County is located in the central and western parts of Hainan Island, covering the wild areas of Wuzhishan Mountain and the northwest foot of Limushan Mountain. It has steep terrain, and high mountains. This county used to be a malaria-endemic county in Hainan Province. From 2005 to 2010 (Fu et al., 2014), 49.6% of malaria cases in Baisha County were indigenous cases of *P. vivax* malaria, and 2.1% were indigenous cases of *P. falciparum* malaria. Due to the natural forests of Baisha County, a forestry company employed a large number of people as migrant forest goers to carry out tree planting and logging in the mountain forests every year. Approximately 18% of sporadic indigenous malaria cases of *P. vivax* have originated from this forestry company each year since 2005. Most of these cases were male workers under the age of 30. The following strategies were implemented to accommodate for the increasing challenge of higher mobility in forest goers (Cai et al., 2009). (1) Passive case detection (PCD) and active case detection (ACD) of malaria in forest goers was improved. In 2003, a network report system for reporting infectious diseases was established in Baisha County. All records from every hospital in Baisha could be reported in real time in this network, including all forest goer cases. For all reported malaria cases, personal information (including patient address) and type of malaria infection were collected and shared with Baisha CDC staff to implement ACD. From 2005 to 2010, 52 forest goer cases were confirmed at the forestry company, and ACD was subsequently carried out in each focus. (2) Outbreak thresholds were updated. The threshold was defined as (a) two indigenous malaria cases within a month in an administrative village where no indigenous malaria cases had been reported at the township level for 3 consecutive years or (b) more than five indigenous malaria cases reported within a month in an administrative village where indigenous malaria cases had been reported in townships for 3 consecutive years (Cai et al., 2009). (3) Timely files for each sporadic case were established to ensure on-site treatment of the epidemic. Case information, epidemic investigation information, and blood tests were recorded, chemoprophylaxis was administered to known contacts of confirmed cases in forest goers, and vector surveillance and control (IRS or distribution of LLNts or ITNts) information and health education were recorded and analysed in a timely manner (Fig. 15).

3.3 Transmission patterns and interventions in the elimination stage: A retrospective study on outbreaks in forest goers

In 2015, an outbreak of 6 total *P. malariae* cases in forest goers occurred in Sanya City (Lin et al., 2016). This outbreak originated with an indigenous

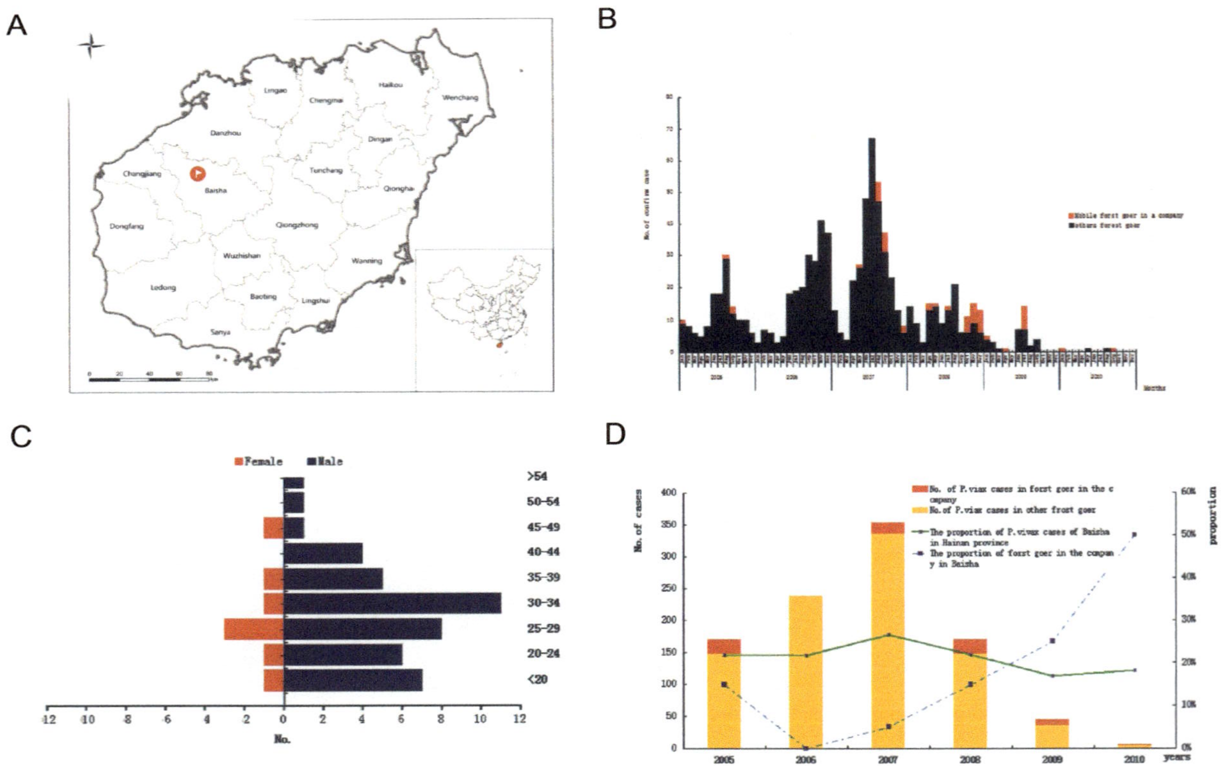

Fig. 15 Surveillance and response of sporadic malaria in forest goers in Baisha County (A. Location of Baisha County in Hainan; B. Sporadic case of *P. vivax* in forest goers in Baisha from 2005 to 2010; C. Distributions of *P. vivax* by age and sex in forest goers from the company from 2005 to 2010; and D. Changes in the proportion of *P. vivax* cases in forest goers from the company from 2005 to 2010).

case of *P. malariae* that was unexpectedly detected in a hospital in Sanya. According to the 1-3-7 approach, ACD was performed with guidance from information from Case 1. Cases 2–4 had the same epidemiological history as Case 1 and were similarly confirmed to be infected with *P. malariae*. Case 1, who worked with Cases 2–4, overnighted in the mountains to collect bodhi fruit. These four cases had a history of overnighting in the mountains before the onset of fever and were thus classified as forest goers. However, the clues from Case1 came to an end and it was uncertain whether there were other potential infection sources or whether transmission was established in local villages. Case screening in these villages was decided to be the most effective way to solve this dilemma. A detailed three-layer strategy (TLS) that integrated malaria joint prevention and control strategies (JPCSs; one of Hainan's important public health policies since 1992) with the 1-3-7 approach was implemented. Gaofeng township is located at the edge of Sanya city, bordering Baoting and Ledong County and Wuzhishan City.

In view of the geographical location of malaria cases, villages with cases and adjacent villages were regarded as the first layer in the prevention and control strategy. Gaofeng Town with cases and adjacent towns were regarded as the second layer. Sanya city with cases and adjacent counties or cities were regarded as the third layer (Fig. 16). In the rapid response and screening stage, the detailed strategies were as described below.

Three villages in Gaofeng Town in Sanya city and seven villages in Xinzheng Town of Baoting County were included as the first layer of the TLS. In this layer, active case detection (ACD) was mainly carried out in the villages of foci and their surrounding villages. To improve detection accuracy, polymerase chain reaction (PCR) was carried out on dried blood spots and other suspected samples to detect parasites in the first layer. The partial SSU rRNA gene was amplified by PCR with Plasmodium-specific primers (rPLU1 and rPLU5) in Nest1 PCR and genus-specific primers (rPLU3 and rPLU4) in Nest2 PCR (Li et al., 2013). A total of 1823 blood slides were examined by microscopy, and blood spots from residents in 10 villages in Baoting and Sanya were screened by PCR. Three positive samples were found from slide samples, and 13 positive samples were found by PCR of blood samples on filter paper. After cross-checking, four cases were identified. Case 4 and Case 6 were neighbours, but Case 6 had no history of being a forest goer. Case 5 presented with similar symptoms and sought medical treatment voluntarily. Case 5, who worked with two other individuals, had an similar epidemic history with Case 1. However, the two co-workers of Case 5 were negative for malaria.

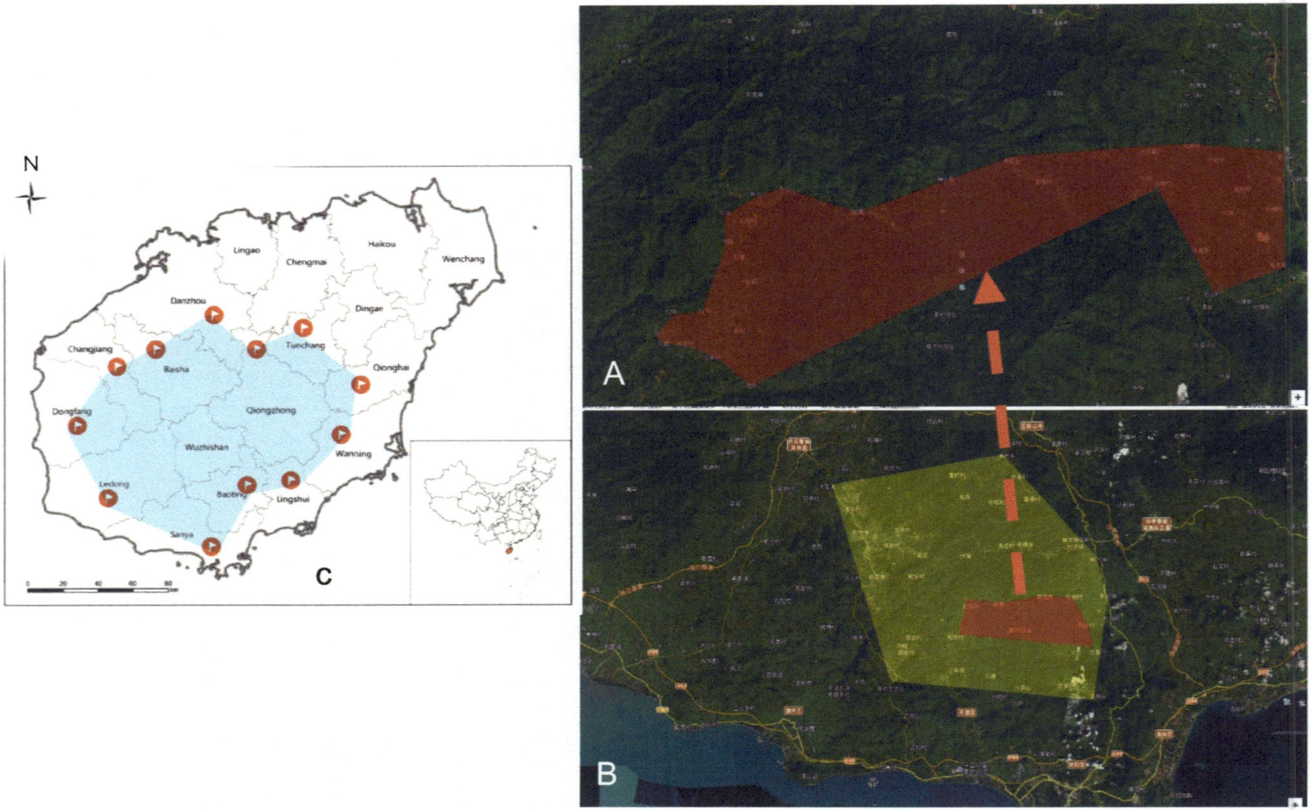

Fig. 16 The TLS, which integrated malaria JPCSs and the 1-3-7 approach, was applied to the outbreak in Sanya in 2015 and used to improve epidemic measures to prevent emergence of residual foci from 2016 to 2018 (A. The first layer; B. The second layer; and C. The third layer).

Meanwhile, vector surveillance and control were carried out to support foci elimination and to minimize the possibility of transmission. *An. minimus*, *An. dirus* and *An. sinensis* were found in the first-layer. IRS was implemented at each foci and long-lasting mosquito nets were distributed to residents. To effectively control this outbreak, Sanya also implemented health education for residents and reminded local villagers to avoid overnighting in the mountains in the future (Fig. 17). Health education, vector surveillance and distribution of long-lasting mosquito nets among forest goers were also carried out in Baoting County (Table 6).

In the second layer of the TLS, 10 townships were included, and passive case detection (PCD) and active case detection (ACD) among forest goers were carried out in Gaofeng townships of foci and surrounding townships, including Gaofeng and Yucai in Sanya City; Daan and Zhizhong in Ledong County; Xiangshui, Maogan, Nanlin, Sandao, and Xinzhen in Baoting County; and Changhao in Wuzhishan City. Forest goers were the main target of PCD and ACD. An emphasis was placed on spot visits to forest goers

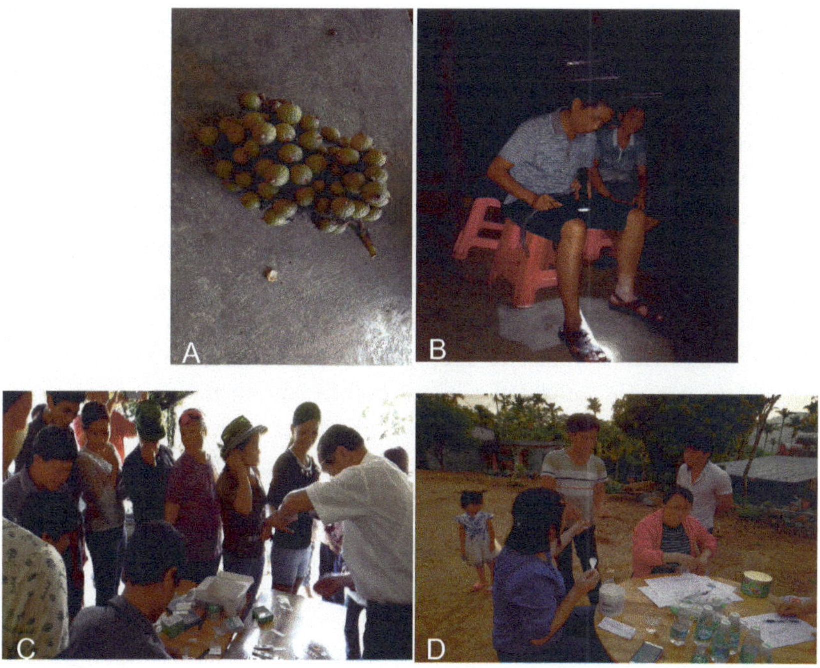

Fig. 17 Epidemic response for forest goers under the TLS in 2015. (A) Bodhi fruit; (B) People used as bait for vector surveillance in 2015; (C) ACD of malaria in 2015; and (D) MDA to prevent malaria from 2016 to 2018.

in the targeted townships and blood slide screening for malaria in forest goers who had a history of overnighting in the mountains as well as fever cases. A total of 7831 slides from all forest goers were screened by microscopy from the target townships.

In the third layer of the TLS, 12 counties or cities were selected for health education, and passive case detection was mainly carried out for forest goers around Sanya and associated counties, including Ledong, Baoting, Wuzhishan Dongfang, Lingshui, Qiongzhong, Baisha, Changjiang, Wanning, Qionghai, Tunchang and Danzhou. The target population was still forest goers. PCD and health education were implemented to alert them to the risks of malaria infections when overnighting in the mountains and to remind doctors to pay attention to malaria symptoms in forest goers. Over 95,350 blood slides from all forest goers were screened in the target townships. *An. minimus* and *An. dirus* were captured in Wuzhishan, Changjiang, Danzhou and Tunchang, but *An. sinensis* was the dominant malaria vector. Long-lasting mosquito nets were distributed to forest goers in 84% of these cities and counties, and clinicians, doctors and laboratory technicians were trained in 92% of these cities and counties.

To achieve the goal of eliminating malaria in 2020, the three-layer strategy (TLS) was also implemented to improve epidemic measures to prevent the emergence of residual foci. The TLS with chemoprophylaxis was adopted for 3 consecutive years from 2016 to 2018. The improved epidemic measures mainly focused on chemoprophylaxis and ACD in forest goers. Piperaquine phosphate was selected as the chemoprophylactic drug. From March 2016 to March 2018, adult residents were given a total dose of 1200 mg piperaquine phosphate orally before bed from 2016 to 2018. Adult forest goer were orally administered 600 mg daily before bed. Doses for children were modified according to their weight and age. Villagers, including forest goers, were required to provide informed consent before administration. At the same time, active case detection (ACD) was carried out in forest goers (Table 5). If fever was found in a forest goer, malaria examination by microscopy was required.

In the first layer, chemoprophylaxis and ACD were carried out in all residents in villages of foci and their surrounding villages; 89.5% residents accepted chemoprophylaxis from 2016 to 2018. In the second layer, chemoprophylaxis and ACD in forest goers were mainly carried out in townships of foci and their surrounding townships. Of the 5489 forest goers in the second layer, 79.1% received chemoprophylaxis. In the third layer, preventive medication and health education were carried out in Sanya and associated

Table 5 The three-layer strategy implemented in response to the 2015 outbreak, and improved intervention measures from 2016 to 2018. (TLS)

			Epidemic response in 2015		Improved measures from 2016 to 2018			
Name of county or city	Name of township	Layer	PCD	ACD	MPD	ACD in FG	CP	%
Sanya	Gaofeng	1st	176 (1)	1642 (4)	398	2113	1825	86.4%
	Gaofeng	2nd	1216	0	1414	0	0	0
	Yucai	2nd	1109	553	2930	1297	1265	97.5%
	others	3rd	11,039	15	28,184	0	0	
Baoting	Xinzheng	1st	320	181	1118	1013	974	96.2%
	Xinzheng	2nd	742	0	1779	707	707	100.0%
	Xiangshui	2nd	331	103	1420	415	375	90.4%
	Maogan	2nd	350	0	1551	1381	341	24.7%
	Nanlin	2nd	600	258	2043	478	478	100.0%
	Sandao	2nd	740		1743	427	414	97.0%
	others	3rd	5529	142	17,579	0	0	0
Ledong	Daan	2nd	83	317	1648	5	5	100.0%
	Zhizhong	2nd	548	32	2080	378	375	99.2%
	Baoguo	2nd	82	447	1585	30	24	80.0%
	others	3rd	4261	4332	25,567	191	178	93.2%

Continued

Table 5 The three-layer strategy implemented in response to the 2015 outbreak, and improved intervention measures from 2016 to 2018.—cont'd
(TLS)

			Epidemic response in 2015		Improved measures from 2016 to 2018			
Name of county or city	**Name of township**	**Layer**	**PCD**	**ACD**	**MPD**	**ACD in FG**	**CP**	**%**
Wuzhishan	Changhao	2nd	320	0	1063	371	360	97.0%
	others	3rd	2120	885	8453	726	712	98.1%
Lingshui	–	3rd	5359	1747	22,069	833	808	97.0%
Qiongzhong	–	3rd	3427	2640	18,664	427	425	99.5%
Baisha	–	3rd	6828	588	21,061	207	207	100.0%
Changjiang	–	3rd	2294	2923	15,732	1418	1417	99.9%
Waning	–	3rd	9354	1115	43,330	3732	3366	90.2%
Qionghai	–	3rd	5582	1624	22,376	2016	1952	96.8%
Tunchang	–	3rd	1969	1626	10,219	0	0	0
Danzhou	–	3rd	10,297	158	112,400	325	319	98.2%
Dongfang	–	3rd	9496	0	28,525	489	473	96.7%
Total	–	–	84,172	21,328	394,931	18,979	17,000	89.6%

The numbers in brackets represent the number of positive cases.
MPD: malaria parasite detection; FG: forest goer; CP: chemoprevention; ACD: active case detection; and PCD: passive case detection.

counties for forest goers. Of the 10,364 forest goers in the third layer, 89.6% received chemoprophylaxis from 2016 to 2018.

Vector monitoring and control measures continued from 2015 to 2018. *An. dirus* and *An. minimus* could still be captured in some counties. A total of 385 *An. dirus* and 156 *An. minimus* were captured from 2015 to 2018, but *An. sinensis* was still the dominant species. In addition, long-lasting mosquito nets were distributed to forest goers, except those in Wanning (Table 6). Training of clinicians, doctors and laboratory staff continued from 2015 to 2018 (Table 7).

This case study in Hainan shows that the TLS was effective for eliminating or controlling malaria transmitted by *An. dirus* and *An. minimus* in tropical areas. TLSs combined with the 1-3-7 approach may be an alternative strategy in China's malaria elimination phase. TLSs may be more suitable than the 1-3-7 approach for halting outbreaks, especially outbreaks of indigenous cases from unknown causes.

3.4 Imported cases and surveillance in the elimination stage: 2011–20

From 2011 to 2020, 88 imported malaria cases, including deaths, were reported in Hainan Province (Fig. 18). All imported cases were confirmed in the laboratory, consisting not only of *P. falciparum* and *P. vivax* but also *P. ovale* and *P. malariae*. Cases were reported in 14 cities or counties, but not in Baoting County, Lingshui County, Wuzhishan City or Changjiang County. Haikou City, Wanning City and Danzhou city had the highest number of cases.

Among the reported cases of imported malaria in Hainan Province from 2011 to 2020, there were more cases in males than females; most patients were 18–60 years old and were migrant workers. The 88 imported malaria cases were from 24 countries on three continents: 78.4% from Africa (including Nigeria, Mozambique and Liberia) and 20.6% were from Asia (including Cambodia, Myanmar and Indonesia). During the malaria elimination phase, two case studies on retransmission demonstrate the measures of disposal of imported malaria foci. In Case Study III, the disposal of active malaria foci is illustrated, and species results have been rechecked by PCR since 2012. Case Study IV illustrates the cooperation with customs for case detection, transport, and treatment in isolation, and foci from isolated sites during the COVID-19 epidemic were identified as foci of impossible transmission.

Table 6 Vector surveillance and control from 2015 to 2018.

Name of county or city	Vector surveillance																Vector control[a]			
	2015				2016				2017				2018				No. of distribution in LLNts			
	An. minus	*An. dirus*	*An. sinensis*	others	*An. minus*	*An. dirus*	*An. sinensis*	others	*An. minus*	*An. dirus*	*An. sinensis*	others	*An. minus*	*An. dirus*	*An. sinensis*	others	2015	2016	2017	2018
Sanya	1	0	154	2337	1	2	368	50	0	0	548	140	0	0	187	136	300	1648	598	490
Ledong	0	0	164	283	0	0	182	143	0	0	105	60	0	0	83	30	447	325	165	113
Baoting	0	0	0	15	0	0	319	204	0	0	131	352	0	0	9	15	600	1700	0	0
Wuzhishan	2	18	74	29	2	19	49	5	0	34	10	2	2	21	21	7	600	1000	0	0
Dongfang	0	0	92	296	0	0	11	85	0	0	181	423	0	0	207	1178	700	500	0	0
Lingshui	0	0	95	273	0	0	241	802	0	0	236	675	0	0	88	420	409	670	0	495
Qiongzhong	0	0	357	226	0	0	119	17	0	0	61	16	0	0	36	2	600	700	0	0
Baisha	3	19	910	1126	9	0	242	409	0	0	418	126	1	0	224	48	600	700	0	0
Changjiang	100	0	327	1137	0	40	116	268	1	3	93	212	1	0	9	124	1564	424	309	134
Wanning	0	0	97	214	0	0	116	164	0	0	94	154	0	0	65	146	0	0	0	0
Qionghai	0	0	0	0	1	0	663	185	1	0	107	312	23	0	53	261	2610	2409	1415	0
Tunchang	17	0	1249	2927	9	0	1081	3647	19	0	2253	3110	0	0	470	177	0	300	0	0
Danzhou	154	0	73	11	37	0	124	154	1	0	108	10	0	0	120	0	300	300	0	60
Total	277	37	3592	8874	59	61	3631	6133	22	37	4345	5592	27	21	1572	2544	8730	10,676	2487	1292

[a]The IRS data are not shown; IRS was implemented only in Sanya for disposal of six foci.

Table 7 Training personnel in 13 counties or cities for malaria detection and intervention from 2015 to 2018.

	Clinicians				Doctors				Laboratory technicians			
Name of county or city	**2015**	**2016**	**2017**	**2018**	**2015**	**2016**	**2017**	**2018**	**2015**	**2016**	**2017**	**2018**
Sanya	23	18	20	24	36	24	20	22	29	18	26	19
Ledong	25	26	46	0	51	68	34	23	25	26	46	23
Baoting	28	23	24	17	83	43	72	20	16	17	19	15
Wuzhishan	9	11	10	0	10	10	10	23	10	10	6	0
Dongfang	24	21	22	27	42	42	22	27	23	21	23	22
Lingshui	21	46	56	22	45	66	56	56	42	25	22	22
Qiongzhong	105	0	25	24	0	0	0	0	2	0	27	4
Baisha	26	85	24	0	42	54	0	0	31	38	26	0
Changjiang	10	16	27	0	21	21	30	33	14	25	30	25
Waning	15	100	24	23	335	190	24	24	0	32	22	20
Qionghai	10	0	73	27	70	60	51	21	34	0	20	17
Tunchang	25	11	19	44	21	20	15	45	18	14	22	38
Danzhou	28	18	17	0	106	34	17	23	47	32	17	0
Total	349	375	387	208	862	632	351	317	291	258	306	205

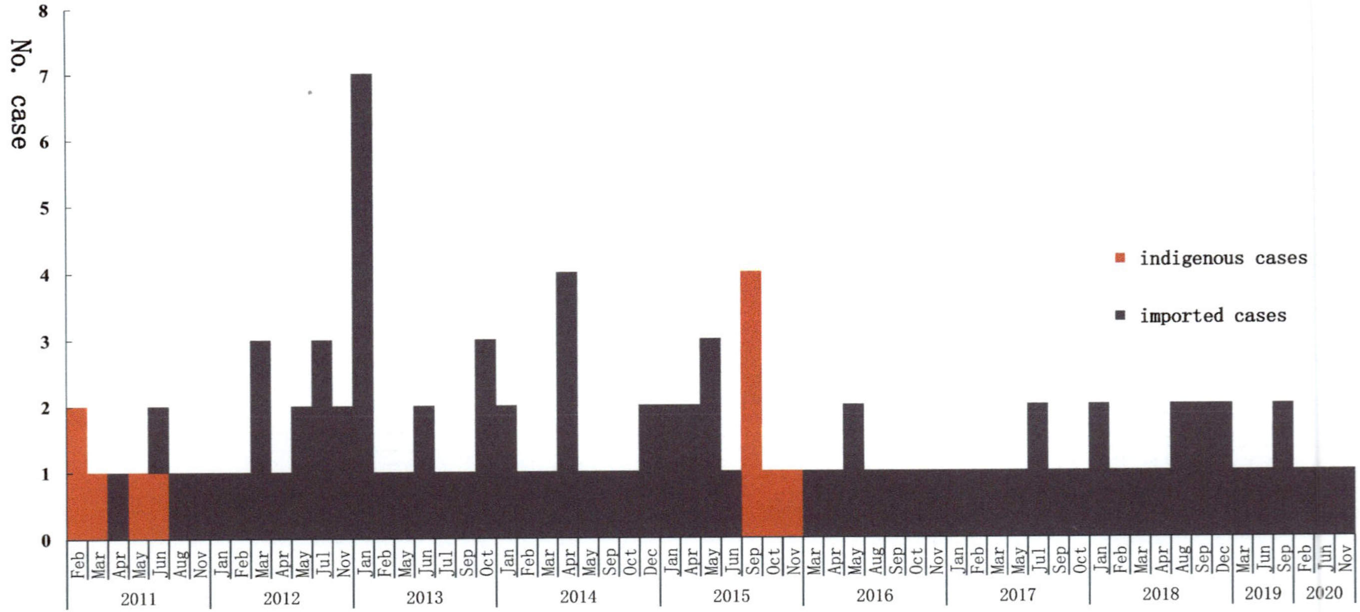

Fig. 18 Imported and indigenous malaria cases from 2011 to 2020.

Case Study III: A positive malaria case in a 49-year-old Chinese male who worked abroad. On February 28, 2013, the patient had symptoms of chills and a fever and went to a township hospital. Blood samples were collected to test for malaria parasites. *P. vivax* was identified and reported on the same day. The patient had gone to Sierra Leone on June 4, 2012, developed symptoms, such as chills and fever, in Ghana in July 2012 and visited a local medical institution; there, he was diagnosed with a cold, but symptoms were alleviated by an injection of artemisinin. He left for China on December 30, 2012, and returned home on January 4, 2013, via Guangzhou and Haikou. The patient had no contact with outsiders before symptom onset and had was no history of blood transfusion within 15 days of onset. There were no fever patients at home and no patients with similar symptoms in the village. The blood samples were examined by the county CDC and the provincial Reference Laboratory for Malaria Diagnosis and PCR testing was conducted. *P. ovale* was identified by microscopy, and *P. ovale wallikeri* was confirmed by PCR (Li et al., 2013). The patient was given radical treatment and cured according to the standard national treatment guidelines. No malaria cases in this location were reported within 5 years. A total of 58 people at the epidemic foci were screened by blood smear, but the results were all negative. *An. sinensis* and other anopheles were captured in the area, but *An. minimus* and *An. dirus* were not captured. Deltamethrin was used to carry out IRS for villages around the epidemic foci, covering an area of 1307 m^2. In addition, health education was provided to the surrounding villagers through the distribution of leaflets and other forms. After being cured, the patient underwent a blood test once a week, three times in total, and was followed-up at 3, 6, 9 and 12 months after cure. Blood samples were collected for malaria testing and were negative.

Case Study IV: A positive malaria case in a 29-year-old Chinese male from Jilin Province that worked abroad as construction worker. The patient departed from the Democratic Republic of the Congo on June 9, 2020 and reached Sanya on the same day. His body temperature was normal at entry. An epidemiological investigation was carried out at Haikou Customs when the patient reported that he had been diagnosed with malaria 3 days before his entry. He went to the Democratic Republic of the Congo in October 2017 to work and had been diagnosed with malaria several times over the past 3 years. In view of the COVID-19 quarantine, he was transferred to a designated hotel in Sanya that served as an isolated site for centralized medical observation, and blood samples were collected and sent to Haikou Customs for malaria testing. On June 12, 2020, *P. falciparum* was identified by microscopy. He was admitted to Naval Hospital, given dihydroartemisinic piperaquine tablets, and had recovered by June 18. Moreover, his blood samples were rechecked by the Sanya CDC on June 13 and the Hainan Provincial Reference Laboratory for Malaria Diagnosis on June 16; *P. falciparum* was confirmed. The other individuals who returned to China with this patient tested negative for malaria.

4. Ongoing challenges and responses in forest goers after malaria elimination in Hainan Province

4.1 Challenges in forest goers after malaria elimination in Hainan Province

Hainan is building a China free trade port and will therefore have an increasing number of highly mobile international travellers (Wang, 2021). Increased mobility in populations will increase malaria cases.

4.1.1 Surveillance in both forest goers and migrant populations

Health surveillance of forest goers is an ongoing challenge, especially after the elimination of malaria. Forest goers infected with malaria can include both local forest goers and migrants, as well as tourists. In recent years, cities and counties in the central forest region of Hainan have also vigorously developed resources for ecological tourism and rural tourism (Shi, 2021). Tourists enjoy travelling in mountain forest areas (Li, 2020). The maintenance of malaria surveillance, including forest goers' attitude, knowledge, behaviour and living environment, is a new challenge.

4.1.2 Maintaining a rapid response mechanism to prevent reintroduction of malaria

The management and prevention of malaria retransmission among migrant and tourist forest goers are new challenges. Migrant and tourist forest goers will be difficult to track because of their high mobility. Moreover, there are highly effective malaria vectors in mountainous areas. Four types of malaria from imported cases have been found, and the retransmission of malaria from imported malaria cases is highly probable.

4.1.3 Alarming super-long latent cases in forest goers

P. vivax is mainly prevalent in the local mountain population, but long-term latent cases and residual cases among local residents are easily overlooked

(Zhu et al., 2008). These long incubation periods may cause a new round of transmission in Hainan due to the presence of highly effective malaria vectors (Kim et al., 2013).

4.2 Response in forest goers to malaria elimination in Hainan Province

Forest goers will still be the susceptible to malaria and are important in preventing the retransmission of malaria; tourists may also join this group, although an updated TLS approach has been developed to respond to outbreaks and eliminate malaria. *An. dirus* and *An. minimus* are still the main malaria vectors. Due to the prevalence of these vectors, it is very likely that indigenous cases of malaria will be introduced from imported cases.

4.2.1 Constant surveillance of malaria cases and vectors

Passive surveillance of fever patients should be carried out monthly, and active surveillance of forest goers should be carried out every year. Blood from fever patients should be tested, and the mobile population should be the focus of attention. Moreover, malaria vector surveillance should be maintained and improved.

4.2.2 Training and QA activity

Malaria diagnostic laboratories in hospitals at various levels are equipped for conducting malaria microscopy and rapid diagnosis tests (RDTs). Each city or county CDC has at least one qualified microscopist to identify positive slides and distinguish *P. falciparum* malaria and non-*P. falciparum* malaria from positive slides. Remote areas that have no capacity for microscopy are equipped with RDTs to facilitate rapid diagnosis of malaria by local doctors. Continuous training must be conducted to reduce the impact of staff turnover.

4.2.3 Improving treatment and cooperation from authorities

Professional technical institutions should continue to keep clinicians vigilant in malaria diagnosis and treatment, improve multisectoral cooperation, and share information resources. In particular, the hospital treatment for severe *P. falciparum* malaria should be maintained and improved.

Acknowledgements

We thank all researchers, medical workers, government workers and local community members who have been involved in malaria control and elimination in the Hainan forest goers over the past 30 years. Moreover, we thank Prof. Xiaonong Zhou and Dr Jianhai Yin from the National Institute of Parasitic Diseases, Chinese Centre for Disease Control and Prevention (Chinese Centre for Tropical Diseases Research) for their help during the preparation and writing of this manuscript. This work was supported by the Bill & Melinda Gates Foundation (No. INV-018913) and the Hainan Provincial Basic and Applied Basic Research Program (Natural Science Foundation) for High-level Talents in 2019 (2019RC394) and Natural Science Foundation of China (No. 81460520).

References

Baoting and Lingshui Sanitary and Epidemic Control Station and Hainan Island Institute of Tropical Disease Control, 1962. Summary of Malaria Eradication Work in Lingshui and Lingshui Counties in Baoting in 1958, Malaria Data Album of Hainan Island (1953–1959).

Cai, X.Z., 1993. Forty years of malaria control in Hainan. Hainan Med. 3, 1–3.

Cai, H., Cai, Z., 1996. Analysis of sources of malaria infection in 10 malaria control pilot areas in Hainan Province. Hainan Med. 2, 65–66.

Cai, Z., Cai, H., 1998. Analysis of malaria infection of mobile population among 10 poilt bases in Hainan province. Hainan Med. 2, 78–79.

Cai, X., Zhang, H., Pang, X., Zeng, Q., Chen, W., Wang, X., Wu, Z., Huang, Q., Liu, D., Wu, D., 1984. Investigation on the resistance to chloroquine falciparum malaria in Hainan Island. Hainan Health 2, 5–10.

Cai, X., Liang, Z., Si, Y., Li, Y., 1990a. Effects of deltamethrin-impregnated mosquito nets and DDT indoor residual spraying on the control of malaria focal points carried by Anopheles minimus. Hainan Med. J. 3, 6–8.

Cai, X., Liang, Z., Wang, Y., 1990b. Effects of deltamethrin impregnated mosquito nets on anopheles dirus. J. Parasitol. Parasitol. Dis. 4, 72.

Cai, K.N., Wang, G.C., Fu, X.Z., Liang, Y.M., 2009. Malaria infection among mobile population in Baisha county, Hainan Province in 2007. Chin. J. Trop. Med. 9, 905.

Chen, W., Shi, P., Wu, K., Deng, D., Tang, L., Cai, X., Gu, Z., Si, Y., Lin, M., Yan, W., 1995. Impact of socio-economic factors on malaria prevalence in Hainan province by unconditional Logistic multiple regression analysis. Chin. J. Parasit. Dis. 3, 161–164.

Chen, W., Wu, K., Lin, M., Tang, L., Gu, Z., Wang, S., Changxiong, L., Lan, X., Li, H., Huang, M., Chen, X., Sheng, H., 1999. Pilot study on the control of malaria in mountainous areas of Hainan by strengthening the prevention and control of infectious sources combined with health education. Chin. J. Parasitol. Parasitosis 1, 4–7.

Chen, W., Wu, K., Lin, M., Li, C., 2007. Great achievements and technical problems of malaria control in Hainan Island in half a century. Chin. J. Trop. Med. 7, 2013–2017.

Duan, J., Zhang, Y., Liang, H., Chen, G., Zhu, M., 1999. Control of an outbreak of plasmodium vivax malaria in Qiongzhong County. Chin. J. Parasitol. Parasitol. Dis. 5, 16.

Edwards, H.M., Canavati, S.E., Rang, C., Ly, P., Sovannaroth, S., Canier, L., Khim, N., Menard, D., Ashton, R.A., Meek, S.R., Roca-Feltrer, A., 2015. Novel cross-border approaches to optimise identification of asymptomatic and artemisinin-resistant plasmodium infection in mobile populations crossing Cambodian borders. PLoS One 10, e0124300.

Fu, S., Wang, J., Fu, X., Wang, G., 2014. Analysis of the results of global fund malaria project in Baisha County, Hainan Province from 2003 to 2012. Chin. J. Trop. Med. 14, 1288–1290.

Gao, H., 2009. September 1. People's Hainan 60 Years: a vow to drive malaria out of Qiongzhou. Hainan Daily A6.

Hainan Institute of Tropical Disease Control, 2000. Compilation of Malaria Control Data in Hainan Province (1984–1999).

Hainan Island District Party Committee Leading Group Office of Disease Eradication, 1962. Malaria Prevalence and Epidemic Factors in Hainan Island. Malaria Data from Hainan Island (1953–1959).
He, Q., 1956. Significance of eliminating anopheles minimus. In: Department of Health and Epidemic Prevention, Ministry of Health of the People's Republic of China, National Professional Conference on Malaria Control Data Compilation.
He, Q., 1965. Research on malaria in new China. Chin. Med. J. (Engl.) 8, 491–497.
He, Q., Deng, D., Qian, H., 1964. Continuing Investigation on the Distribution of *Anopheles minimus* in Hainan Island. Annual Report of Institute of Parasitic Diseases, Chinese Academy of Medical Sciences.
He, Y.J., Huang, R.J., Ji, W.Q., Liu, S., 1993. Investigation and analysis of an outbreak of P. vivax malaria in Xinxing Miao Village. Hainan Med. J. 2, 3–4.
He, C., Wang, S., Hu, X., Wang, G., Huang, C., 2012. Analysis of malaria associated KAP in shangshan li ethnic population of Dongfang city, Hainan province. Chin. J. Public Health 28, 525–526.
Hewitt, S.E., 2019. Let's 'cut to the chase' on malaria elimination in the Greater Mekong Subregion. Trans. R. Soc. Trop. Med. Hyg. 113, 161–162.
Institute of Parasitic Diseases of Hainan Administrative Region, 1985. Prevalence of Malaria in Hainan Island, Malaria Control Research Data in Hainan Island (1950–1983). pp. P2–120.
Kim, S.J., Kim, S.H., Jo, S.N., Gwack, J., Youn, S.K., Jang, J.Y., 2013. The long and short incubation periods of Plasmodium vivax malaria in Korea: the characteristics and relating factors. Infect. Chemother. 45, 184–193.
Li, S., 1997. Research status of Anopheles minimus in Hainan Island. Hainan Med. 2, 69–71.
Li, L., 2020. Study on Spatial-Temporal Pattern and Influencing Factors of Inbound Tourism in Hainan Province. Hainan Normal University.
Li, S., Zeng, L., Liang, Q., 1990. Investigation on DDT resistance of Anopheles dirus in Hainan. Hainan Med. 3, 140.
Li, Y., Wang, G., Sun, D., Meng, F., Lin, S., Hu, X., Wang, S., 2013. A case of Plasmodium ovale wallikeri infection in a Chinese worker returning from West Africa. Korean J. Parasitol. 51, 557–562.
Lin, M., Li, H., 1999. Study on the antimalarial effect of deltamethrin impregnated mosquito net in high malaria mountainous area. Chin. J. Public Health 5, 22.
Lin, M., Weng, S., 2013. Progress on malaria control in 60 years in Nanqiao Pilot project and progress in the implementation of global fund projects against malaria. Chin. J. Trop. Med. 13, 245–248.
Lin, M., Chen, S., Deng, J., Si, Y., Zhong, H., Huang, M., Chen, X., Cao, R., 1993. Investigation on malaria infection among residents of FOREST GOERS accommodation in high malaria area of Hainan Province. Hainan Med. J. 4, 8–9.
Lin, M., Chen, S., Deng, J., Si, Y., Zhong, H., Chen, W., Huang, M., Chen, X., 1994. Investigation on malaria infection among mountain residents living in high malaria mountainous area of Hainan Province. Chin. J. Parasit. Dis. 1, 71.
Lin, C., He, Y., Tang, D., Ji, W., 2000. Surveillance of Anopheles dirus in high malaria area of Hainan province from 1990 to 1994. Chin. J. Parasit. Dis. 1, 10–12.
Lin, M., Wenjiang, C., Shanqing, W., Gu, Z., Li, H., Lan, X., 2001. Effects of health education on malaria control. Chin. Health Educ. 3, 9–11.
Lin, C., Lin, S., Fu, Z., Ji, W., Li, H., 2005. Investigation and analysis of malaria control among FOREST GOERS population in malaria area of Ledong County. Chin. J. Trop. Med. 2, 257–335.
Lin, M., Wu, K., Chen, W., 2009. Epidemiological analysis of focus malaria outbreaks in anopheles minimus in Hainan island. China. Chin. J. Trop. Med. 9, 805–806.

Lin, C., Chen, Z., Wang, S., Luo, P., Wu, D., Zheng, A., Wei, J., 2016. Analysis and management of a rare malaria case of P. malariae in Sanya, Hainan province. Chin. J. Trop. Med. 16, 481–484.

Liu, Y., 1957. Malaria Control Experiment of Overseas Chinese Collective Farm in Hainan. Annual Report of Institute of Parasitic Diseases. Chinese Academy of Preventive Medicine.

Liu, Y., 1960. Malaria Eradication Research Institute in Beida Town, Hainan Island. Institute of Parasitic Diseases, Chinese Academy of Preventive Medical Sciences 1960 Annual Report.

Ma, C., 2010. Malaria incidence has been basically controlled in Our province. Hainan Daily A02.

Ma, K., 2021. China has been Certified by WHO to Eliminate Malaria, and Hainan is One of the Four Provinces to be Certified On-Site. Hainan Daily B06.

Pan, B., 2003. Morphological characteristics, ecological habits and role of major malaria vectors in China. J. Trop. Med. 4, 477–480.

Sheng, B.L., 1957. Investigation of Natural Infection of Vectors in Hainan Island. Institute of Parasitic Diseases.

Shi, X., 2021. Measurement and evaluation of tourism ecological coupling degree under the construction of Hainan Free Trade Port. China Bus. Theory 20, 40–42.

Si, Y., Pang, X., Chen, W., Zhong, H., Cai, H., 1992. Malaria epidemiology in Hainan in 1991. Hainan Med. 4, 6–8.

Si, Y., Cai, X., Chen, W., Pang, X., Zhong, H., Cai, Z., 1993. Effect of deltamethrin impregnated mosquito net on mosquito control and malaria in Hainan Province. J. Pract. Parasit. Dis. 4, 24–26.

Si, Y., Zhong, H., Pang, X., 1994. Analysis of malaria infection among mobile population in Hainan province from 1990 to 1992. Hainan Med. J. 5, 8–10.

Si, Y., Pang, X., Cai, H., Lin, C., Liang, Z., Kong, X., Su, A., Fu, J., Chen, S., 1995. A case study of malaria outbreak in Dashichang, Changliu, Haikou city. Hainan Med. 1, 1–2.

Si, Y., Pang, X., Du, J., He, Y., Wang, G., Cai, Z., Lan, C., Lin, S., 1998. Effect of pilot malaria control in Hainan province. Chin. J. Parasit. Dis. 2, 3–5.

Su, S., Wang, Z., He, G., Wang, S., Lin, Q., Chen, H., Lin, H., Huang, R., Ji, W., 1985. Experimental observation on the spread of Anopheles dirus in Hainan Island. Parasitol. Parasitol. Dis. 2, 36–38.

Sun, D.W., Du, J.W., Wang, G.Z., Li, Y.C., He, C.H., Xue, R.D., Wang, S.Q., Hu, X.M., 2015. A cost-effectiveness analysis of Plasmodium falciparum malaria elimination in Hainan Province, 2002-2012. Am. J. Trop. Med. Hyg. 93, 1240–1248.

Sun, D., Li, y., Wang, G., Wang, S., 2016. Mid-term evaluation report of action plan for malaria elimination in Hainan province. China J. Trop. Med. 16, 338–342.

Tang, L., Lenore, M., Deng, D., Wu, K., Cai, X., Lan, C., Gu, Z., Wang, K.A., 1995. Social aspects of malaria in Heping, Hainan. Acta Trop. 59, 41.

Wang, G.Z., 1997. Investigation on sources of malaria infection in Hainan province from 1990 to 1995. Prev. Med. Lit. Inf. 2, 110–111.

Wang, S.Q., 2019. The seventy years of malaria from hyperendemicity to elimination in Hainan. Chin. J. Trop. Med. 19, 707–718.

Wang, L., 2021. Benchmarking and learning from the experience of world-class free trade ports to promote the high-quality development of Hainan Free trade Port. Bankers 9, 4–5.

Wang, G.C., Kai-Ning, C., Liang, C.Y., Fu, Y.Q., Chen, C., Chen, J.-H., 1998. Investigation and analysis of sources of malaria infection in Baisha County, Hainan Province from 1987 to 1996. Hainan Med. J. 1, 4–5.

Wang, G.M., He, Y.J., Tang, D.H., Wu, D.L., Cai, B., Ji, W.Q., Wang, G.-Y., 2002. Malaria control strategies and measures in Heping Malaria control base of Hainan Province. Chin. J. Parasit. Dis. 5, 9–11.

Wang, G., Wang, S.Q., Hu, X.M., Zhu, Q.X., Zeng, W., Cai, H.L., Li, Y.C., Meng, F., 2013. Analysis of effectiveness of malaria joint control in 20 years in Hainan province. Chin. J. Trop. Med. 13, 1339–1342.

Wei, S., Lin, S., Yang, C., 2007. The 50-Year History of Health Service Development in Hainan Province from 1950 to 2000. Nanfang Press, Haikou.

Wen, S.Q., Luo, P.W., Feng, Y.M., Zhong, C.L., Fu, G.L., 1997. Effect analysis of malaria control test in Dongfang district, Dongfang County, Hainan. Hainan Med. J. 2, 74–76.

Wu, C., 1960. Efficacy of Primaquelin in Linwang Area of Hainan Island. Annual Report of Institute of Parasitic Diseases. Chinese Academy of Preventive Medical Sciences.

Wu, K., Chen, W., Tang, L., Deng, D., Lin, M., Cai, X., Pan, Y., Gu, Z., Yan, W., Huang, M., Zhu, W., Sheng, H., Chen, X., 1995. Study on the characteristics of lodging behavior and its relationship with malaria infection among Li and Miao ethnic groups in high malaria mountainous area of Hainan Province. Chin. J. Parasitol. Parasitosis 4, 17–21.

Wu, K., Tang, L., Chen, W., Liu, D., Lin, M., Gu, Z., Lan, C., He, Y., Wang, Z., Chen, G., Cai, X., Deng, D., 1998. Epidemiological characteristics of malaria in mountainous areas of Hainan. Chin. J. Parasit. Dis. 4, 3–7.

Wu, D., Wang, G., Tang, D., Wang, G., Wang, S., 2001. Effects of naphthoquine phosphate on the control of malaria in Qiongzhong County, Hainan province. Chin. J. Trop. Med. 3, 216–217.

Xia, Z.G., Xu, J.F., Zhang, S.S., Wang, R.B., Qian, Y.J., Zhou, S.S., Yang, W.Z., Zhou, X.N., 2014. The analysis of the intervention measures of malaria from control to eliminate. Chin. J. Schistosomiasis Prev. Control 26, 598–601.

Xu, Y., 2014. Evaluation of Malaria Control Programs Fudan University. Fudan University.

Xu, J., Qu, F., 1997. Study on the taxonomic status of Anopheles dirus from Hainan province using rDNA. Chin. J. Parasitol. Parasit. Dis. 5, 15–18.

Zeng, X.L., 2015. Distribution Characteristics and Environmental Factors of Malaria in Hainan. Third Military Medical University.

Zhan, M., 2006. Investigation report of an outbreak of imported Falciparum malaria. Pract. Prev. Med. 1, 110.

Zhang, L., Feng, J., Zhang, S.S., Xia, Z., Zhou, S.S., 2016. Analysis of malaria epidemic in China in 2015. Chin. J. Parasitol. Parasitosis 34, 477–481.

Zhou, Z., 1957. Study on Ecological Habits of Four Anopheles Species in Eastern Hainan Island. Institute of Parasitic Diseases, Chinese Academy of Preventive Medical Sciences.

Zhou, Y.C., 1980. Observation on a outbreak of malaria newly infected in mountain and its control effect. Hainan Health 1, 54–56.

Zhu, Q.-X., 2002. Investigation and management of a malaria spot outbreak among mobile population in Hainan Mountain forest area. Chin. J. Trop. Med. 2, 239–241.

Zhu, D., Yang, W., Wang, J., 2008. Research progress on the long incubation period of plasmodium vivax. Chin. J. Epidemiol. 1, 81–84.

CHAPTER FOUR

Mass drug administration in response to vivax malaria resurgence in Anhui Province of Huanghuai Plain, China

Xian Xu, Jian-Jun Wang, Jing-Jing Jiang, Tao Zhang, Xiao-Feng Lv, Shu-Qi Wang, Zi-Jian Liu, Wei-Dong Li*, and Xue-Chun Lu
Anhui Provincial Center for Disease Control and Prevention, Anhui, PR China
*Corresponding author: e-mail address: ahcdclwd@126.com

Contents

1. Introduction 116
2. Background 117
   2.1 Malaria transmission patterns in Anhui Province 117
   2.2 Outbreak of vivax malaria and responses in Anhui Province from January 2000 to June 2007 118
3. Designing the focal MDA 121
   3.1 Determination of the scope of fMDA 121
   3.2 Design the other technical issues of focal MDA 130
4. Implementation of focal MDA 133
   4.1 Preparations before MDA 133
   4.2 fMDA implementation 135
5. Other malaria control measures 141
   5.1 Formulation of the goals for malaria control 142
   5.2 Improving the competency of case finding 142
   5.3 Strengthen timely and standardized treatment and case reporting 142
   5.4 Vector control 142
6. Effectiveness of the response to the resurgence 144
   6.1 Malaria situation after taking medicine 144
   6.2 Malaria diagnosis competency deficiency 146
7. Conclusions and perspectives 147
   7.1 Conclusions 147
   7.2 Perspectives 148
Acknowledgements 149
References 150

Advances in Parasitology, Volume 116
ISSN 0065-308X
https://doi.org/10.1016/bs.apar.2022.04.001

Abstract

This article summarizes the background, specific conditions, main measures, steps and effects of the implementation of Mass Drug Administration (MDA) to control the local *P. vivax* malaria epidemic in Anhui Province in central China. Distributing medicines to the designated population quickly controlled the local epidemic of *P. vivax*. Implementing MDA to control *P. vivax* ensured the correct selection of medicines, clarification of the targeted population for receipt of medicines, and assurance of a high rate of compliance through government support and health education. These results provide a reference for countries and regions experiencing similar events and planning to implement MDA in malaria control.

1. Introduction

Malaria remains at the top of the global burden of diseases. According to World Malaria Report 2021, an estimated 241 million malaria cases occurred in 2020 globally, and 627,000 people died. Malaria remains the disease with the highest morbidity and mortality in most parts of the world (World Health Organization, 2021). The World Health Organization (WHO) set a goal to eliminate malaria in at least 35 countries by 2030. However, many countries are still trying to bring malaria outbreaks under control. China was certified malaria-free by the WHO on June 30, 2021, after persistent efforts through the national malaria control and elimination programme for seven decades in the country. While in the pre-elimination stage of the national malaria control programme from 2000 to 2010, the resurgence of *P. vivax* malaria occurred in central China including Anhui Province remain the major challenges for malaria elimination, due to its predominant distribution in the country and complexity in the lifecycle of the *P. vivax* parasite that relapses frequently occurred because of hypnozoites activation and become a new source of transmission, even after the schizonts of *P. vivax* are cleared from the blood. While, successfully fighting a resurgence of *P. vivax* from 2000 to 2007 in Anhui Province, located in the eastern part of China. At that time, the province had the largest number of cases and the highest incidence rate in the country. Among the four common *Plasmodium* species that infect humans, *P. vivax* was the most widely distributed in the country. To extinguish the resurgence, a drug-based intervention, namely, the Mass Drug Administration (MDA) (Nadia and Lu, 2022), was used to eliminate the source of infection from 2007 to 2015 among the several key populations in Anhui Province. MDA laid a solid foundation for achieving malaria elimination. This article summarizes the lessons on MDA implementation and its effects in coping with the relapse of malaria in Anhui Province and provides a reference for countries and regions experiencing similar events.

2. Background

2.1 Malaria transmission patterns in Anhui Province

Anhui Province located in the eastern part of China (Fig. 1) between 114° 54′E-119°37′E and 29°41′N-34°38′N， with an area of 140,100 km^2. There are over 16 prefecture-level cities, 61 counties (cities), 44 county-level districts, and 1509 townships in Anhui, with a total resident population of 61.05 million at the end of 2020 (Chen and Liu, 2021). Anhui Province is in a transition zone of warm temperate and subtropical climate zones. Two important rivers, the Yangtze River and the Huaihe River, flow

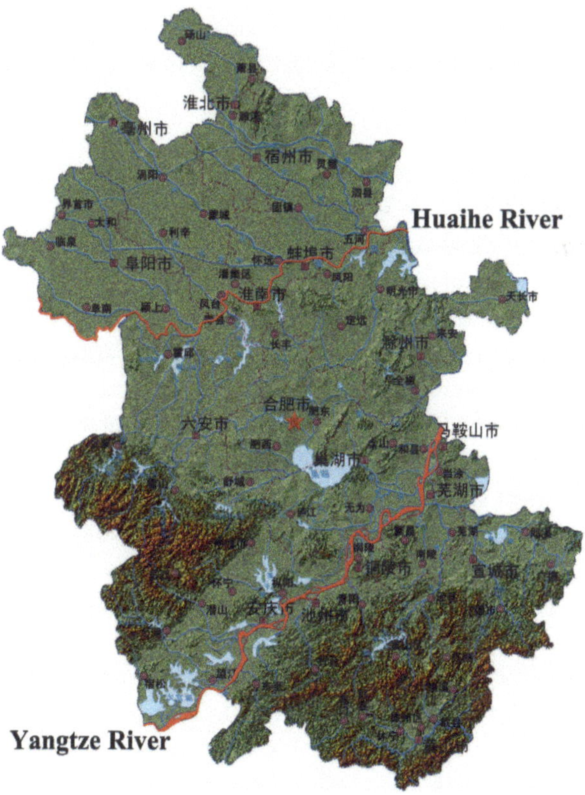

Fig. 1 Administrative division of Anhui Province.

eastward across the south and the north of the province, respectively, dividing its area into three natural regions (Fig. 1). The province has a warm temperate semi humid monsoon climate to the north of the Huaihe River and a subtropical humid monsoon climate to the south of the Huaihe River. The annual average temperature is 14–17 °C, and the average precipitation is 800–1800 mm. Historically, malaria was usually transmitted between May and October.

Anhui Province is one of the historically key malaria-endemic provinces in the country, where *P. vivax* was the dominant species, followed by *P. falciparum* and a few cases of *P. malariae* (Xu et al., 2020). Anopheles sinensis is the dominant malaria vector and is distributed in areas consistent with the epidemic range of *P. vivax* in the province. Moreover, Anopheles sinensis was the only malaria vector in the Huaibei Plain. The other Anopheles species of Anopheles anthropophagus found in Anhuifrom 1958 to 1999 (Yuan et al., 1991; Shen et al., 1998; Zou et al., 2000; Jiang et al., 2020), was mostly distributed in mountainous and hilly areas in the Huaihe River Basin and most areas to its south, and it was closely related to the transmission of *P. falciparum* (Yuan et al., 1990; Pan, 2003).

2.2 Outbreak of vivax malaria and responses in Anhui Province from January 2000 to June 2007

2.2.1 Resurgence of vivax malaria

In 1970, the incidence of malaria in Anhui Province reached 12,150/100,000. The outbreak was mainly caused by *P. vivax*. Fortunately, it was controlled gradually by measures such as MDA for the key populations during the dormant stage and vector control. Since 1991, no local cases of falciparum malaria have been found in Anhui, and the incidence of malaria had dropped to approximately 0.13/10,000 in 1999 (Xu et al., 2020). See Fig. 2.

Factors such as socioeconomic development, environmental changes, urbanization (Xu et al., 2017), and population mobility (Zhao et al., 2020; Murta et al., 2021) may affect the spread of malaria. From 1999 to 2006, due to changes in the biological barriers caused by the reduction of livestock in rural areas and other factors, including insufficient prevention and control of malaria and the inability to remove the source of infection in a timely manner (Xu et al., 2003; Shen, 2006), the incidence of vivax malaria continued to rise in Anhui Province (Liu, 2007). By 2006, there were 34,984 cases reported, which ranked the province highest in China with an incidence rate of 57.2/100,000 (Fig. 3) (Xu et al., 2015; Zhou

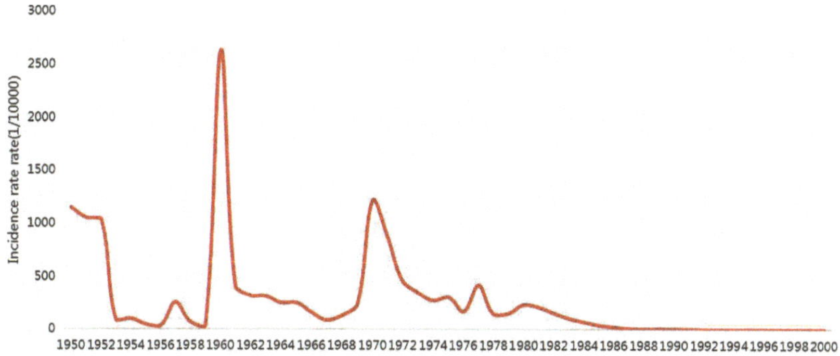

Fig. 2 Malaria incidence in Anhui Province, 1950–2000.

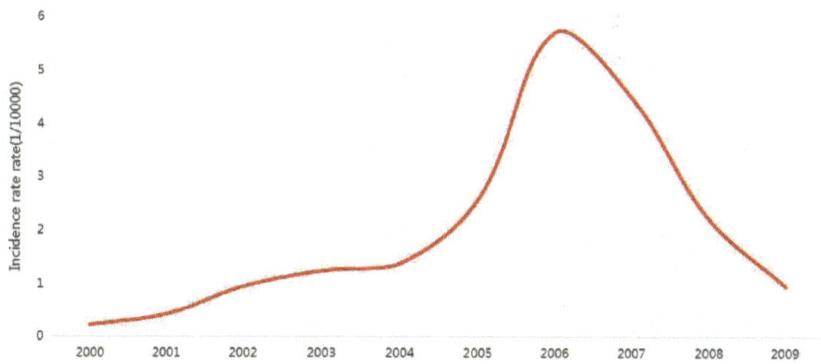

Fig. 3 Malaria incidence in Anhui Province, 2000–2009.

et al., 2007). These cases were mainly distributed in rural parts of 24 counties in 6 cities, including Bozhou and Huaibei, on the Huaibei Plain (Xu et al., 2015) (Fig. 4).

2.2.2 Response to malaria outbreak by MDA

MDA has been a powerful and effective measure to control temperate vivax malaria in China as was the treatment of infected patients. MDA has been widely used in malaria-endemic areas in central and southern China and the provinces bordering Southeast Asia, and it has played an important role in taking China through the stages of high prevalence to elimination (Xia et al., 2014; Zhu et al., 2011; Xu et al., 2017). In terms of implementation time, MDA can be implemented during the malaria transmission season (seasonal malaria chemoprevention, SMC) or before the start of the transmission season (ACCESS-SMC Partnership, 2020). SMC involves the use of a certain antimalarial drug or combination provided intermittently to prevent the occurrence of malaria by maintaining the level of the

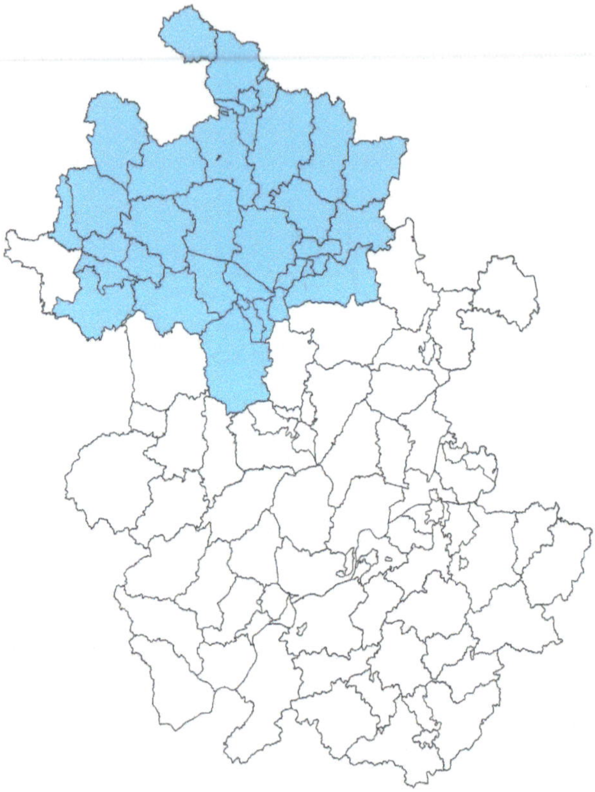

Fig. 4 Geographical location of 24 counties with a high incidence of malaria in Anhui Province in 2006.

therapeutic drug in the blood of the population (Brady et al., 2017) to reduce the risk of malaria transmission during the transmission season. It is suitable for various malaria parasitic infections. The antimalarials are usually *P. vivax* or *P. ovale* infections, which are used in combination with drugs that treat Plasmodium in the blood and liver to achieve complete cure of the patient. This combination of medicines is usually given in winter or spring to prevents cases from entering the transmission season as a source of infection. In terms of the scope of implementation, MDA can be implemented for risk populations or whole populations (all residents of a geographic area or community) such as villages, towns, counties, cities, or provinces (Finn et al., 2020a, b). This practice is implemented worldwide, targeting key populations is called focal MDA (fMDA) and refers to a smaller range of coverage, such as natural villages (Hsiang et al., 2013) or a specific population, such as the implementation in Africa for the family members of individuals who test positive for malaria via the malaria Rapid Diagnostic Test (RDT) (Finn et al., 2020a,b; Bennett et al., 2020), children aged 3–59 months (ACCESS-SMC Partnership, 2020), border residents who travel to and from countries with different prevalence levels (Zhao et al., 2020), and individuals in Henan Province, who take medicines to prevent blood donor transmissions, and their family members (Xu et al., 2011). This drug protocol can also be implemented in some households in which only some members need to take medication.

From January 2000 to June 2007, MDA in Anhui Province was implemented in natural villages before the start of the transmission season. If the incidence rate did not reach 1%, 2% or 3% in the previous year, medications were distributed to individuals who were diagnosed with malaria in the previous year and their family members and neighbours, suspected cases, and others with fevers of unknown origin. If the rate reached 1%, 2% or 3% in the previous year, medications were distributed to the whole population of natural villages, and the medication regimen was the three-day chloroquine phosphate(CP) combined with eight-day primaquine phosphate (PQ). The number of MDA cases before the start of the transmission season was 10,9270, 65,398 and 129,424 in 2005, 2006 and 2007, respectively, and the number of cases in the previous year was 8,912, 15,693 and 34,984, respectively. The number of MDA cases was 12.26, 4.17, and 3.70 times the number of cases in the previous year, respectively.

3. Designing the focal MDA

From 2006 to 2009, the program of fMDA in Anhui Province was reviewed. While it had been the most important measure taken in malaria prevention and control in response to the outbreak of *P. vivax*, research and pilot projects were developed to address technical issues, including the scope of fMDA and type of medication.

3.1 Determination of the scope of fMDA

Anhui Province has implemented fMDA during and before the transmission season since June 2007.The scope of fMDA was determined by factors, including mosquito breeding water bodies and the number of cases. The scope can be a part of a natural village, the entire natural village, or two or several adjacent natural villages; coverage is not limited to administrative boundaries, and medications are administered to everyone within the prescribed area (Zhu, et al., 2007; Zhu, et al., 2013).

3.1.1 Scope determination process

Determining the scope of fMDA implementation based on the spatial distribution of the *P. vivax* malaria outbreak.

Since the prevalent *P. vivax* found in Anhui Province belongs to the temperate type, it has the characteristics of a long incubation period and an intra-hepatic phase because there is no means to detect the intra-hepatic phase of Plasmodium. At the same time, due to the high proportion of asymptomatic infections in the endemic areas of *P. vivax*, there is also a submicroscopic blood level of *P. vivax* (Liu et al., 2018). The detection threshold is much lower than that of *P. falciparum*; thus, it is more difficult to find cases of *P. vivax* than *Plasmodium falciparum*. Further, *P. vivax* is prone to recurrence, and patients are not easily cured. Therefore, MDA needs to be implemented to kill undiscovered or residual malaria parasites in the human body to eliminate the source of infection.

What are the distribution characteristics of malaria cases in a natural village? In 2006, Anhui Province conducted a study on the spatial distribution of malaria cases in 5 counties with a high incidence of malaria cases and selected 5 natural villages in each county for investigation (Fig. 5) (Wang et al., 2006). The actual malaria cases in 2004, 2005 and 2006 were obtained through field visits to all villages, and the Geographic Position System(GPS) was used to record the outlines of the residences, water bodies and natural villages of all malaria cases from 2004 to 2006. The median distance from the cases to the closest mosquito breeding places was 44.20 m. The median distances from the cases in 2004, 2005 and 2006 to the closest mosquito breeding places were 53.85 m, 45.60 m and 43.15 m, respectively. The ratio of the distance from cases to mosquito breeding places in different stratifications is displayed in Fig. 6. The distribution of cases, mosquito breeding places and outline of the natural village are displayed in Fig. 7. Black lines indicate the outline of the natural village. Blue areas and yellow areas represent mosquito breeding places. The former had water all the year. The latter had water only in the transmission seasons. Black dots indicate the residences with malaria cases.

From the results above, it was concluded that most cases surrounded mosquito breeding places and were relatively distributed in natural villages. The results indicated that mosquito breeding places had a great influence on malaria case distribution. The results suggest that we should determine the

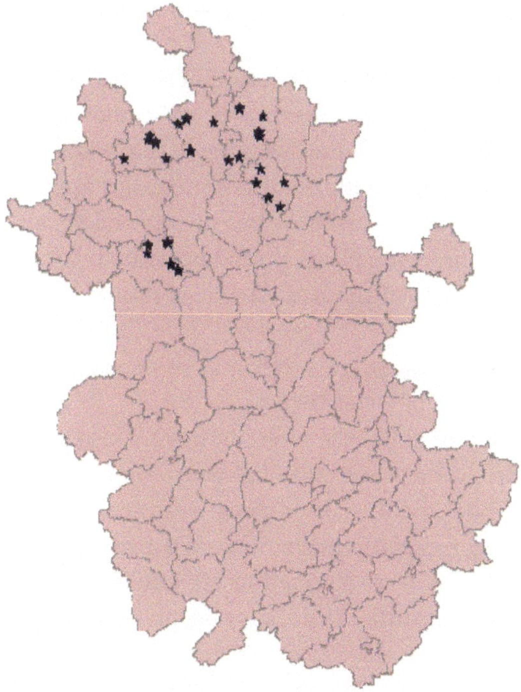

Fig. 5 The investigation site for research on the spatial distribution characteristics of malaria in Anhui Province.

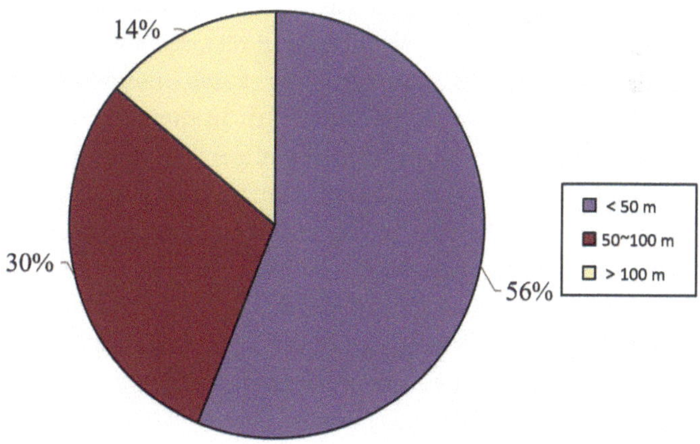

Fig. 6 Ratio of distance from case to the closest mosquito breeding places.

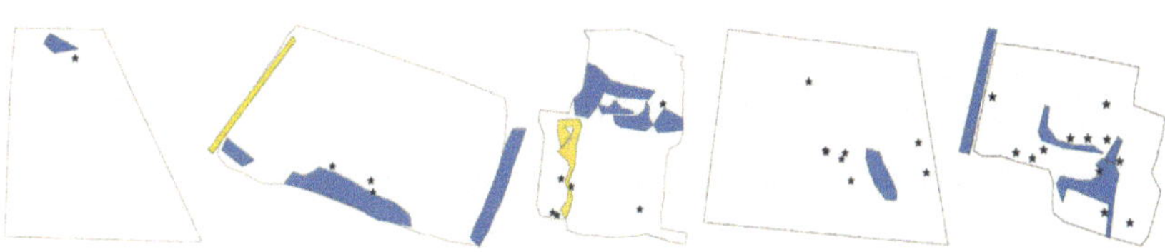

Fig. 7 Geographic position of a natural village with cases in a natural village (1) 1 case, (2) 3 cases, (3) 6 cases, (4) 7 cases, and (5) 12 cases (Wang et al., 2006).

scope of fMDA relative to the distribution of mosquito breeding places and malaria cases. If we only treat malaria cases, we cannot remove all sources of infection in a natural village. Thus, we suggest that when there are 1–3 cases in a natural village, people within 50 m of mosquito breeding places should be treated, and when there are 4–9 cases in a natural village, people within 100 m of mosquito breeding places should be treated. When there are more than 10 cases, all people in the natural village should be treated.

3.1.1.1 Comparison of the effect of fMDA in combination with and without the distribution of water bodies

From April to May of 2007, the effect of fMDA in combination with and without the distribution of water bodies were compared (Zhu et al., 2013). In 30 natural villages, field trials of three treatment methods were carried out. Method 1: All residents within 50 m of the nearest water body associated with malaria cases were selected to take medicine; for natural villages with 4 to 9 malaria cases in 1 village, all residents within 100 m of the nearest water body from 2004 to 2006 were chosen to take medicine; for 1 village with more than 10 patients, the whole population, including the patients in the natural village, administered them medicine. Method 2: The rest period treatment strategy of the intensified antimalarial campaign was approved by the Ministry of Health. This method was designated for natural villages with an incidence rate of $\geq$1% in 2006. The drug recipients were those with a history of malaria within 1 year and their family members, as well as suspected malaria and unknown fever patients. In the natural villages with an incidence rate of less than 1% in 2006, the subjects who took the medicine were those who had a history of malaria within the past year. The above two methods administered three-days of CQ followed by 8 days of PQ. Method 3: The final method used subjects as a control group for comparison with the previous two groups. No interventions were supplied to the selected natural villages during the rest period, and the incidence rates were observed.

The results of the three methods were as follows. The incidence rate in the population using Method 1 was reduced by 16.04%, the incidence using Method 2 was reduced by 7.97%, and the incidence using Method 3 was reduced by 2.54%. There was a significant difference in the change in the incidence rate between Method 1 and Method 3 ($\chi^2=7.74$, $P<0.05$), and there was no significant difference in the change in the incidence rate between Method 2 and Method 3 ($\chi^2=3.69$, $P>0.05$). Compared with the nonintervention group, the PR and IE of Method 1 were 84.2% and 6.31, respectively, while the capture rate was 69.2% (9/13). The conclusion was that delimiting preventive medicine treatment during the rest period of malaria was very effective in eliminating the potential infection source of malaria and reducing the morbidity.

3.1.1.2 Field trial of fMDA in Longshan Town

From April to May 2007, delineation of the risk range of malaria transmission and the drug administration trial were carried out in 101 natural villages in Longshan Town, Guoyang County, which had the largest number of cases in Anhui Province at that time. For delineated groups of people to take medicine, the delineation method was the same as Method 1. The drug regimen was chlorine for 8 days of therapy. The results showed that the number of cases in the town increased by 62.3% in the month and a half after taking the medication compared with the same period during the previous year, but the number of cases in other towns in the county increased by 363.6% during the same period. Moreover, a total of 497 cases of malaria were reported in 2007, a decrease of 39.61% compared with the 823 cases during the same period the previous year.

3.1.1.3 Field trial of fMDA in Yongqiao County

In 2008 and 2009, Yongqiao County was selected as the site of MDA research on malaria control models for Anopheles sinensis in Anhui Province. (Wang et al., 2009).The selection of individuals to be medicated was based on malaria cases in the previous 3 years and the location of bodies of water in natural villages. A model of "$Y = 36.844 + 19.791X1 + 56.359X2$"was used to determine the targeted population and the amount of medicine and human resources needed. Y was the number of people who should take medicine, X1 was the total number of malaria cases in the natural village in the past 3 years, and X2 was the measure of proximity to a body of water; the number of households within 50 m of a water body accounted for the composition ratio of the number of households in the village ($<30\% = 0$).The number of households within 50 m of the water body accounted for the composition ratio of the total number of households in the village ($\geq 30\% = 1$). The specific groups of people taking the medicine were residents within 50 m of a malaria case and within 50 m of the water body within 50 m of the case. The cost of implementing the medication for key groups was 62% lower than that of implementing the universal medication model.

3.1.2 How to determine the range of fMDA

The method of delineating the scope of fMDA in Anhui Province has been continuously adjusted with the development of the above trials and has gone through the following stages.

3.1.2.1 Field trial on fMDA in Suixi County

From July 12 to 19, 2007, Anhui Province selected Suixi County, Huaibei City, an area with high malaria incidence, for fMDA in natural villages with malaria incidence >1% in 2006 and/or 2007. Defining the scope of fMDA was determined as follows: (1) Map the distribution of cases in the natural village in the past 3 years; (2) If there were widely dispersed cases in the natural village, the whole population was included; (3) If the cases were distributed unevenly in a certain natural village, coverage was based on the distribution of cases and the distribution of water bodies.

A total of 91,164 people took medicine in mid-July. Then, the incidence of malaria gradually decreased. Compared with the same period in 2006, the ten-day incidence was +269.8%, +187.10% and −2.6% in early-July, mid-July and late-July, respectively. In late July, the number of cases decreased rapidly. This shows that fMDA was effective in controlling malaria.

3.1.2.2 Implementation of fMDA in 24 counties

In August, September and October 2007, three rounds of piperaquine phosphate were administered in 24 county-level areas along Huaibei for malaria control in Anhui Province (Anhui Provincial Department of Health, 2007). This activity involved natural villages with malaria incidence rates greater than 1% in 2006 and/or 2007.In the later period, due to the abundance of medicines, the fMDA was expanded to all natural villages with malaria cases in 2006 and/or 2007.The scope of fMDA was delineated according to the distribution of cases and water bodies as it was in Suixi County. The scope of fMDA was divided into two categories with various determinants. Fig. 8 shows the whole natural village scenario. (a) The number of cases is large, and there are cases in all directions (east, west, south, north, and middle) in the natural village; (b) The number of cases is large, and less than 1/4 of the natural village has no cases; (c) Although the number of cases is small, there are cases in all directions in the natural village. Fig. 9 shows the part of the natural villages cenarios. The vast majority of cases are concentrated in a certain part of the natural village, and the range is delineated according to the distribution of cases and water bodies. The delineation

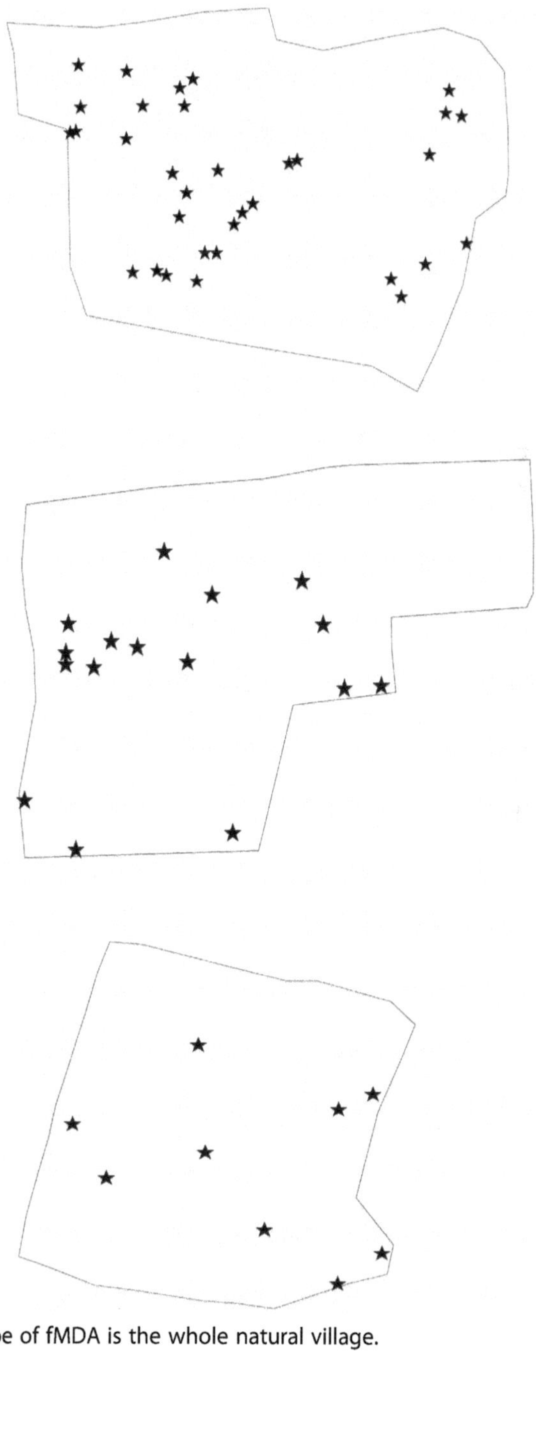

Fig. 8 The scope of fMDA is the whole natural village.

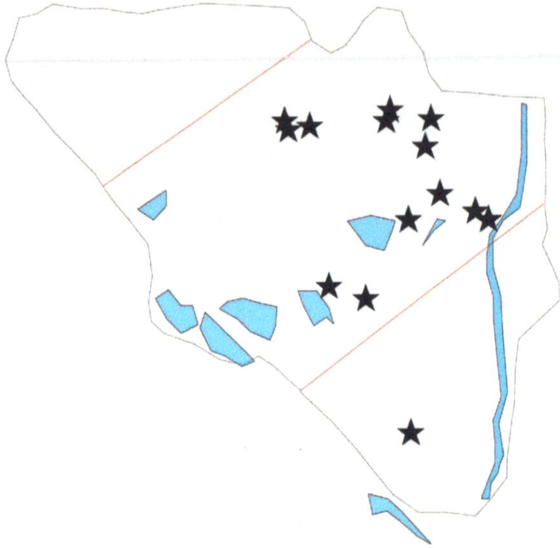

Fig. 9 The scope of fMDA is part of the natural village.

includes most cases and major water bodies. Black lines indicate the outline of the natural village. Blue areas represent mosquito breeding places. Black dots indicate the residences with malaria cases. Red lines indicate the scope of fMDA.

3.1.2.3 Final determination of the method for delineating the scope of MDA

Combined with the test results in Yongqiao District in 2008 and 2009 (Wang et al., 2009), in 2010, Anhui Province finally determined the method for MDA scope delineation (Anhui Provincial Department of Health, 2010). The villages that performed MDA during the malaria cessation period were the natural villages with malaria cases in the previous 2 years. The coverage area was determined by the locations of residences with malaria cases and bodies of water associated with malaria cases in the natural villages in the previous 3 years. The method of delineating the scope of fMDA was as follows: (1) Draw the outline of the residential area in the natural village according to its geographical orientation and mark the main roads to divide the village into sections; (2) Mark the location of all the malaria cases in the village in the past 3 years; (3) If there were widely dispersed cases in the natural village, the scope should be the whole natural village; (4) If the cases were distributed in a certain part of the natural village, mark the location of all water bodies in the village and delineate the scope based on the distribution of cases in proximity to the bodies of water. The scope should include all households within 50 m of the case and 50 m from bodies of water within 50 m of the case, although the scope could be expanded as necessary.

Three doses each of piperaquine phosphates were administered to 1.7168 million people in natural villages with a high incidence of malaria in Anhui Province during the 2007 malaria season. From 2008 to 2015, before the malaria season, 4.056 million people in natural villages with reported malaria cases in the previous 2 years were given PQ. A comparison of the number of people taking fMDA from 2007 to 2013 with the number of malaria cases from 2005 to 2015 in Anhui Province (Fig. 10) revealed that the number of people receiving fMDA was 33.9 times, 28.3 times, 23.7 times, 36.3 times, 48.1 times, 82.9 times and 79.4 times the sum of the number of malaria cases in the previous 2 years. and it 49.1 times, 64.6 times, 71.8 times, 119.2 times, 205.7 times, 364.8 times and 1395.3 times the number of malaria cases in the previous year, respectively.

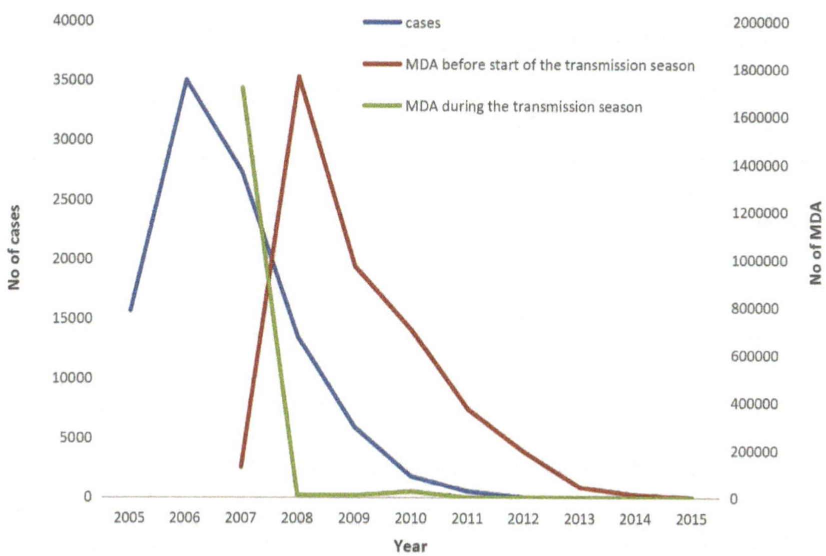

Fig. 10 The relationship between the number of malaria cases and the fMDA medications used in Anhui Province from 2005 to 2015.

3.2 Design the other technical issues of focal MDA

3.2.1 Determination of drugs used in MDA

The drug regimens for prophylactic MDA and radical MDA for vivax malaria were different. With the change in the epidemic situation and the deepening of people's awareness of malaria, the types, dosages, dosing intervals and treatment durations of MDA drugs were different. From 1960 to 1979, the drug used for preventing MDA in China was a regimen of 50 mg pyrimethamine every 10–15 days; the drug used for radical MDA was also the regimen used for clinical and curative treatment: 1200 mg or 1500 mg phosphoric acid CQ for 3 days (600 mg/day 1, 300 mg/day 2–3) + 180 mg PQ for 8 days (22.5 mg/day);in endemic areas, 180 mg PQ for an additional 8 days before the next transmission season was recommended. Thus, the CQ dose for MDA in central and northern China was 1200 mg for 3 days, while it was 1500 mg in Yunnan Province, where transmission intensity was high in remote areas.

From 2000 to 2009, there were two regimens for prophylactic MDA in China: 600 mg piperaquine once a month and 300 mg CQ every 7–10 days. Anhui Province used a regimen of 600 mg piperaquine once a month from August to October 2007. Since 2008, the regimen used for radical MDA in Anhui Province has been changed to a single regimen of 180 mg PQ for 8 days. After 2010, a single regimen of 180 mg PQ was used for both preventive and curative MDA for *P. vivax* throughout China, and it was applied in Anhui, the border areas of Yunnan, and mountainous areas in Hainan to prevent potential malaria epidemics. PQ is the only widely used drug that kills the intra-hepatic dormant body of *P. vivax*, but it has serious side effects (hemolytic anaemia) in patients with G6PD deficiency. The 14-day PQ therapy recommended by the WHO does not completely eliminate dormant *P. vivax*, and the cure rate is usually less than 80%. The radical treatment strategy used in China can completely eliminate *P. vivax*. Since it takes 8 to 14 days of PQ, some scholars have proposed replacing PQ with tafinoquin (Murta et al., 2021), but there has been no report of actual implementation.

3.2.1.1 Determination of piperaquine phosphate

In August, September and October 2007, due to the insufficient supply of PQ nationwide, piperaquine phosphate tablets were used in three rounds of population medication in 24 counties in Anhui Province. The regimen was 4 tablets (base 600 mg) for adults, once a month.

3.2.1.2 Determination of the eight-day PQ

From July 12th to 19th, 2007, the natural villages in Shuangdui Town and Suntuan Town in Suixi County, where the incidence rate was at a middle and then high level, residents took three-day CQ combined with four-day PQ and four-day PQ, respectively. There was no difference in the decrease in malaria cases between the two groups after taking the drug compared with the same period in the previous year ($P > 0.05$) (Table 1).Therefore, province officials decided that from 2008 onward, the three-day CQ combined with eight-day PQ therapy for fMDA was changed to a single eight-day PQ (Table 2).

3.2.2 Determination of medication time

Before 2009, most of the medicines were distributed in April and May during the rest period of malaria in Anhui Province. In 2008, a survey of migrant workers in 20 natural villages in 4 counties, 4 townships and 20 natural villages in Bozhou City (Cheng et al., 2013)showed that the incidence of malaria among those returning home during the busy farming season was higher than that among those who did not return home, and the busy farming season was the season for malaria transmission. Therefore, the time of medicine administration during the rest period of malaria from January to February before and after the Spring Festival in 2009 instead of April to May as in previous years was moved up to cover migrant workers returning home, thereby reducing the incidence of malaria among them and preventing the spread of malaria from other areas with high rates of malaria to areas with low or no malaria.

3.2.3 Determination of the fMDA object

Since 2008, people in the natural villages that were in the malaria cessation period but had malaria cases in the previous 2 years took medicine. The contraindications of taking the drug were as follows: less than 1 year old,

Table 1 Comparison of malaria cases in towns with different medication regimens.

Town	Medication regimen	2006.7.20–2006.10.20	2007.7.20–2007.10.20	±(%)
Shuang Dui	Three-day CQ combined with four-day PQ	279	103	−63.08
Sun Tan	Four-day PQ	358	132	−63.13

Table 2 fMDA dosing schedule used in Anhui from 2007 to 2015.

Age group (year)	Piperaquine Phosphate; number of 600 mg tablets (used in , 2007)	CQ; number of 0.155gtablets (used in 2007)	PQ; number of 7.5 mg tablets (used from 2007 to 2015)
1–3	0.5	1/2 on the first day, 1/4 on the second and third day	1/2
4–6	1	1 on the first day, 1/2 on the second and third day	1
7–9	1.5	1.5 on the first day, 2/3 on the second and third day	1.5
10–12	2	2 on the first day, 1 on the second and third day,	2
13–15	3	3 on the first day, 1.5 on the second and third day	3
16	4	4 on the first day, 2 on the second and third day	4
Times	Once per month for 3 months	Once per day for 3 days	Once per day for 8 days

pregnant women, lactating women, elderly and frail, long-term cardiovascular disease and liver and kidney insufficiency. Since many residents in rural areas worked in other more economically developed regions, such as the surrounding towns and cities, they were excluded from taking the medications.

3.2.4 Determination of medication indicators

To clarify the strategic goals of the malaria campaign, the drug-taking indicators were determined to be the actual drug-taking rate and the whole-process drug-taking rate of the natural villages.

The actual drug-taking rate = the actual number of people taking the medicine/the number of people who should take the medicine * 100%.

The whole-course drug-taking rate = the number of people taking the medicine in the whole process/the actual number of people taking the medicine * 100%.

To ensure the effect of taking the medicine, the actual taking rate should be >90%, and the whole taking rate should be >85%, which was required for the natural village as the unit in 2007 in Anhui Province. Since 2008, both rates have been adjusted to 90%.

4. Implementation of focal MDA

Government leadership and extensive community participation are necessary conditions for the implementation of MDA (Fehr et al., 2021). Medication compliance is related not only to the scope of medication but also to the course of medication selection and delivery methods. It also depends on the local government's support for the implementation plan and the intensity of public propaganda (Keys et al., 2021).

4.1 Preparations before MDA

4.1.1 Government leadership

Strong government leadership guarantees that the population will take medicine. Before the start of the medication every year, the provincial, prefectural, county and township governments held a mobilization meeting and signed a responsibility letter agreeing to the implementation goals in Anhui. In 2007, the provincial government held a special meeting on malaria control key areas along the Huaihe River. The plan to medicate a wider range of people was put forward. The whole province was required to highlight the key points and effectively strengthen the prevention and control of malaria in the Huaihe River region. From 2008 to 2011,health department sat all levels held a special meeting on a similar topic every year and signed an annual responsibility letter.

At the beginning of each year, the county governments held a conference on fMDA attended by the county magistrate, the health bureau, the CDC, the finance bureau, the education bureau, the radio and television bureau, the drug administration bureau, and the heads of the townships and health centres. An administrative group led by government leaders with multidepartment participation was established; the health administrative department established a malaria prevention and control technical guidance group with the director in charge as the team leader and the leaders of the CDC and related professional and technical organizations as members.

This conference established a number of county-level supervisory teams composed of bureau-level cadres, township cadres and professional and technical person neland divided into groups to supervise key towns and towns, find and solve problems in a timely manner; and establish a drug reaction emergency treatment team. The township government and the health centre also set up corresponding leading groups, technical guidance groups and drug reaction treatment groups. Each village established a team composed of township prevention and protection doctors, village cadres, village doctors and other relevant personnel responsible for the thorough investigation, participant registration, delivery of medicines, and compliance supervision.

4.1.2 Funding

To ensure the effective implementation of fMDA, the national-, provincial-municipal- and county-level governments allocated special funds for the purchase of medicines, personnel training and staff subsidies. The Global Fund for malaria control was also involved. In 2007, the Anhui Provincial Government allocated 4.8 million yuan for the special purchase of antimalarial medicines for fMDA during the transmission season. Huaibei City invested more than 800,000 yuan in special funds for malaria prevention and control, and the city organized nearly 4000 people to settle in the villages. Each individual participating in the delineation of the scope of coverage at all levels in the county and village was equipped with pads, pencils, erasers, pencil sharpeners, paper and other tools. In Chenji Town Health Center in Suixi County, rubber shoes and umbrellas were distributed to each drug delivery person, and a subsidy of 100 yuan was provided. In some towns and villages in Lixin County, certain subsidies were provided to relevant personnel, and a certain amount of food as meals (two boxes of yogurt, two pieces of bread, two packs of instant noodles, two bottles of water, two eggs, and two sausages) was provided to each drug delivery person in Suixi County. All of these incentives greatly improved the enthusiasm of the grassroots staff.

4.1.3 Personnel

A medicine delivery team consisting of 3–5 members at least 1 doctor from the health centre, 1 village cadre and 1 village doctor was organized in each natural village participating in the program. It was the key to ensuring the target medication rate. The influential, appealing, and prestigious village doctors and/or village cadres were selected to deliver medicine to improve compliance. In total, more than 15,000 medicine delivery teams were organized for the fMDA in 2007.

4.1.4 Institutional responsibilities

Rewards and punishments were set up according to the assessment and score for the quality of fMDA. Rewards were given to grassroots organizations and individuals who made outstanding contributions. To strengthen the sense of responsibility among village doctors and to link medicine delivery with the interests and welfare of village doctors, economic or administrative penalties were imposed on village doctors who demonstrated a lack of responsibility.

For example, in 2009 and 2010, the Dingyuan County government commended the township governments with outstanding performance in the fMDA work and gave rewards ranging from 1000 yuan to 5000 yuan. In 2009, village doctors who delivered medicines received subsidies in advance, and villages with a large number of fMDA participants were given additional rewards of 3000 yuan, 2000 yuan, and 1000 yuan according to the number of residents taking medicine. Penalties included criticisms in circulars and the withholding of 200–3000 yuan in wages. Other cities imposed penalties on village clinics that refused to carry out fMDA work by revoking their business licences.

4.2 fMDA implementation

The process of MDA implementation should be clear, detailed and comprehensive, and it is necessary to improve the compliance rate through targeted health education through multiple channels, and quality control should be carried out simultaneously. Good planning and implementation are needed, including detailed scheduling, adequate supply of medicines, well-trained staff, and the awareness and participation of target communities (Baba et al., 2020, Fehr et al., 2021, Finn et al., 2020a,b).

4.2.1 Technical training

Centralized training for village doctors and village cadres was critical to the quality of fMDA. The personnel at all levels involved in the plan must be clear about the program requirements and strictly implement them. During the implementation period, 15 resident supervisory teams and 2 tour supervisory teams were organized at the provincial level to inspect and supervise the organization and implementation of fMDA in 24 counties in 2007. The regional government attached great importance to it, convened mobilization and coordination meetings of governments at all levels and relevant departments, and invested enough manpower and material resources to achieve the goals. Before the start of fMDA implementation in 2007, the Provincial Centres for Disease Control and Prevention held a training course on the implementation plan in Anhui Province. Then, 7 groups organized by the Provincial CDC went to 22 key counties to carry out field training on the implementation plan and the method of delineating the scope of medication coverage. Technical guidance teams were set up and carried out staff training before implementation at the provincial, prefectural and county levels. Provincial-level officials conduct face-to-face technical training at the prefect uraland county levels, including delineating the scope of medication coverage, determining the subjects to be administered, identifying contraindications to medication, identifying and treating adverse drug reactions, and filling out medication work forms. At the prefect uraland county levels, professionals were trained to delineate the scope of medication coverage in each natural village and to train the medication teams on medication technology so that personnel at all levels were clear about the program requirements and able to strictly implement them. In the following years, provincial-level training was held at the prefectural level, and township and village staff were then trained at the county level.

4.2.2 Survey and distribution of medicines

Before medicines were distributed, all localities registered the list of people who need to take the medicine and confirmed the number of participants. The number of registered cases is the key to the development of MDA, and the number of cases in each natural village in the previous 3 years must be accurately collected. In addition to checking the medical records, it was also necessary to visit each household to identify some residents that have become ill but have not been diagnosed, some diagnosed but unreported, and some people who became ill but did not seek medical attention.

4.2.3 Publicity

Health education is critical to improve compliance in fMDA implementation. Each participant needs to know why he or she should take medicine, how to take the medicine, and precautions.

First, the local governments held mobilization meetings with different sectors, including health, finance, radio and television, education and other departments. Second, various forms of health education and publicity on the knowledge of malaria prevention and control were organized and tailored to local conditions. These activities could significantly improve compliance. For example, a wealth of publicity materials were produced and distributed, a health education prescription was required for each drug user, and the local malaria prevention and treatment consultation telephone number was published on these materials. Advanced notice about medication distribution was given and informed consent was obtained.

In rural areas, the existing conditions for health education included the following: residents have TVs at home, residential buildings are made of brick or concrete, most buildings were two-story buildings or one-story tile houses, each natural village had a committee and basic clinics, large natural villages had primary schools, and most natural villages were equipped with outdoor loudspeakers. To improve medication compliance, the methods for health education were updated as follows: 1. Publicity was distributed via TV stations, radio stations, newspapers, feature films, and cartoons. 2. Knowledge about malaria prevention and treatment was posted on the walls of buildings, outer walls of the village centre and roadside houses in each natural village; 3. The village chief of the natural village publicized the precautions on the rural broadcasting loudspeaker; 4. A variety of products, such as aprons for home use, calendar pictures, magnetic soft screen doors, shopping bags, eye charts for students, workbooks, and pens also advertised health education.

Table 3 shows some malaria health education products produced and distributed at the provincial level in Anhui Province from 2007 to 2015.

Table 3 Some malaria health education products produced by and distributed in Anhui Province from 2007 to 2015.

Type	Quantity (piece)	Type	Quantity (piece)
Flyer	1,020,000	Discs	30,000
Disposable paper cup	1,000,000	Microscope slide box	40,000
Pen	980,000	Electric mosquito swatter	10,000
Shopping bag	770,000	Microscopic map	10,000
Apron	400,000	Mosquito net	6000
Playing Cards	300,000	Graphics	5000
Eye chart posters	300,000	Panels	1138
Magnetic soft screen door	85,000	Mosquito trap	37
Calendar painting	80,000	Flash animation	1

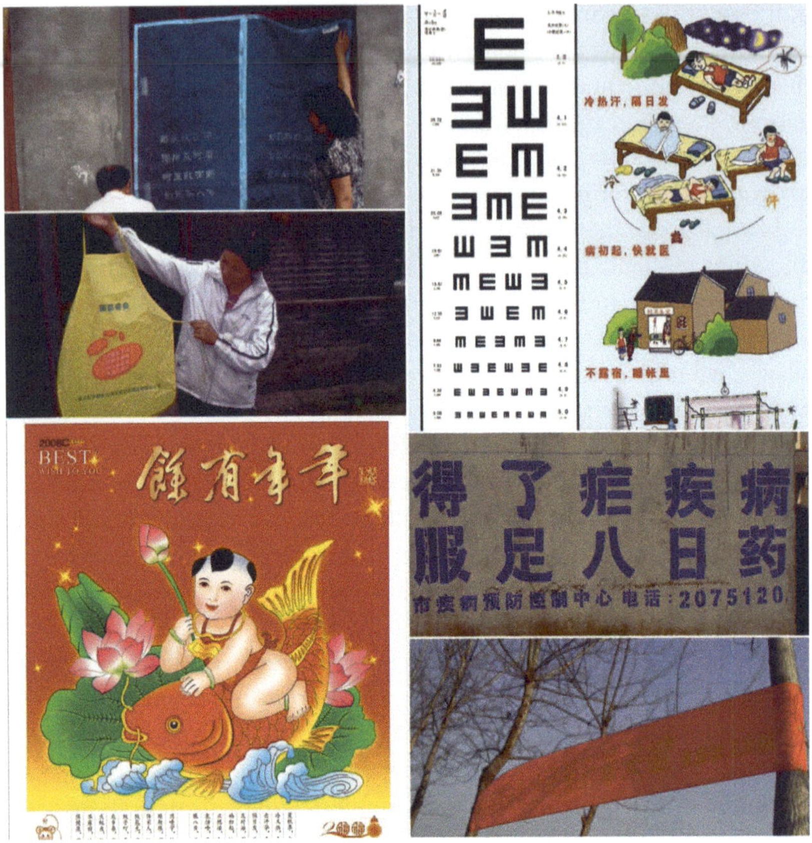
冷热汗，隔日发
病初起，快就医
不露宿，睡帐里
BEST
年年有餘
得了疟疾病
服足八日药
市疾病预防控制中心电话:2075120

Fig. 11 Health education and publicity carried out before and during medication administration in various regions. (11–1 The staff is installing the magnetic soft screen door; 11–2 The apron; 11–3 The calendar posted on the wall of the villagers' houses, printed with a jingle about malaria prevention and control; 11–4 the eye chart posted in the classroom, with Malaria prevention and control pictures and text; 11–5 banners hanging on trees in villages; 11–6 wall slogans painted on the outer walls of villagers' homes).

These funds came from the Global Fund Malaria Program at a total cost of US$777,000. In these products, dialects, parallel sentences, and jingles were used. Some health education products and activities are shown in Fig. 11.

During the fMDA in the 2007 transmission season, various localities adopted the following methods to publicize prevention and control knowledge of malaria symptoms, treatment, and mosquito control to villagers. First, the topic of malaria prevention and control knowledge was disseminated via local TV stations, newspapers and other major media, including films by local people. The malaria prevention propaganda films produced by well-known doctors are broadcast on TV stations and with feature films shown in rural areas. Second, leaflets, propaganda fans, and malaria health education prescriptions are distributed by relevant government departments, township health centres and village clinics, and village committees put up posters. Third, in cooperation with the local education commission, a malaria awareness chart is posted in each classroom of all primary and secondary schools in the project township, and malaria prevention education is taught. The knowledge of malaria prevention and control is then disseminated to parents and neighbours through students. Fourth, a publicity apron is given to each household in natural villages with high rates of malaria. At least 3 walls with slogans are in each village. Administrative villages with a low incidence of disease should have at least 2 posters in each village, and the total number of posters in each township should not be less than 30. In addition, prophylaxis is also good publicity and education. The villagers can acquire certain knowledge of malaria and improve their awareness of timely medical treatment and self-protection.

4.2.4 Antimalarial drug administration

The medicine delivery teams in each village are composed of township doctors, village cadres, and village doctors. They visit residents door to door every day to deliver medicines and directly observed adverse drug reactions, to "deliver the medicine to the hand, take the medicine to the mouth, and do not leave without taking the medicine." This kind of direct supervision treatment method is the DOT method (modified directly observed therapy) (Finn et al., 2020a,b), which promotes the coverage, compliance and safety of the medication. Studies have shown that home delivery and encouragement of staff determine the rate of compliance, and home delivery and face-to-face publicity can effectively increase the acceptance of MDA (Silumbe et al., 2020). MDA should use multiple visits to maximize compliance (Baba et al., 2020).

It is required that the drug-taking rate of the subjects be $>90\%$. Although fMDA is effective in malaria control, for some healthy subjects, there is no direct benefit from the medication, and it may cause drug-related side effects. However, if the malaria parasite is not completely eliminated in the population implementing fMDA, the spread of malaria will continue, and malaria will remain a health risk to the community. Someone may propose screening before taking the drug. However, the limitations of technology, funds and workload make large-scale screening almost impossible

(Liu et al., 2018). The goal of fMDA is to eliminate the malaria parasite in the population. The effectiveness of the medication depends largely on the coverage area, although this may have side effects on individual people. However, the benefits to the community far outweigh the risk of adverse drug reactions in a small number of people (Deng et al., 2018; Keys et al., 2021). The fMDA implemented in China, including mandatory observations, has minimized the potential harm of malaria. Based on community participation, the high rate of compliance can reduce the incidence and even eliminate malaria by eliminating the infection in patients and hosts.

To reduce the occurrence of adverse reactions and avoid gastrointestinal discomfort caused by medicines on an empty stomach, centralized drug delivery for a period of time after breakfast and lunch was implemented in some towns. It is necessary to carry out medication activities after obtaining the review of the ethics committee (Eisele et al., 2020, Finn et al., 2020a,b) and the informed consent of the subjects. A Health Education Prescription was given to each person taking the medicine, and warnings about side effects such as anorexia, epigastric discomfort, vomiting, abdominal pain, cramping, and dizziness were part of the written consent form. Medical institutions at all levels were also used as the adverse reaction disposal units. Severe reactions included cyanosis accompanied by dizziness, chest tightness, palpitations, shortness of breath and other hypoxic symptoms or severe poisoning or allergic reactions. The treatment methods for adverse reactions were provided in advance.

During the 2007 transmission season in 2007, people who had received piperaquine phosphate reported mild side effects, such as dizziness (29.0%), nausea (17.6%), and numbness (10.9%) of the cheeks (10.9%) (Gou et al., 2008). A total of 719 people in the province had serious adverse reactions, but no poisoning or deaths occurred. Likewise, no deaths occurred in the fMDAs before the start of the transmission season from 2008 to 2015.

4.2.5 On-site guidance and supervision

During the implementation of fMDA, health professionals and administrative personnel are responsible for the guidance and supervision of the work of each natural village. The former guides scientifically and rationally delineate the scope of medication and accurately grasp the contraindications and precautions of the technical aspects; the latter is from management. In terms of promoting the population's compliance rate to meet the requirements, methods of supervision included on-site supervision, tour supervision and telephone inquiries. Supervision considerations included being meticulous but also strategic. For example, when asking the subject whether he or she took the medicine, supervisors asked: What colour is the medicine taken? How many slices did you eat? How many days have you taken the medicine? How many pills do you have left? Any problems found during supervision were resolved in a timely manner to ensure the quality of the program.

During the annual fMDA, supervisors are organized at the provincial, municipal and county levels to conduct supervision. The Provincial Department of Health and the Provincial Centres for Disease Control and Prevention organized a number of resident supervisors and several itinerant supervision teams to inspect and supervise the organization and implementation of the program in various counties. The provincial level was in charge of documenting the supervision results at the end of the work every year. The government departments and health departments of all cities and counties have established supervisory groups, and each supervisory group is responsible for its work. The supervision of government departments is very important to increase the emphasis on this work at the township level. For example, the county head in charge of health in Guoyang County supervises onsite at the township and village levels for more than 10 working days during the annual medication period. The bureau-level cadres are in charge of the tablets, a daily summary report during the medication period, and a progress briefing.

4.2.6 Antimalarial drug administration for migrant workers

It was better to deliver medicine when villagers were at home. If they were not at home, the medicine and supervision occurred the next day. Those who left home for long periods of time were required to take their medicines, be aware of the dosage and precautions and be supervised by telephone every day. Alternatively, supervisors could retain the medicines and wait for the migrants to return, then deliver the medicines to their homes.

5. Other malaria control measures

In addition to MDA, the following measures have also been used to strengthen the management of patients and to move forward on the control and elimination of malaria.

5.1 Formulation of the goals for malaria control

The annual goal for malaria control was set up and adjusted according to the malaria situation in different periods. It was required to be reduced by 30% in 2008 compared with the previous year and by 20% in 2009–2011.

5.2 Improving the competency of case finding

Malaria microscopists at the county and township levels in malaria-prone areas were trained every year and ensured the quantity and quality of microscopes for malaria diagnosis at the township level, thereby facilitating the timely diagnosis of malaria cases. From 2000 to 2010, a total of 5.615 million blood tests for Plasmodium were carried out in the province. Since 2012, all towns and villages in the province have been allotted RDT, and a malaria reporting reward system, including subsidies for clinicians and laboratory doctors who diagnosed and treated cases, has been implemented. The subsidy standard was 1000–1500 yuan per case.

5.3 Strengthen timely and standardized treatment and case reporting

Since 2006, antimalarial drugs have been distributed to village-level clinics in key malaria prevention and control counties in Anhui Province. All antimalarial drugs were uniformly purchased at the provincial level and distributed to the municipalities, counties, townships and villages. All levels were registered in the warehouse according to the unified registration book. The village doctor was responsible for supervising the daily medication of each case for 8 days. This ensured that each case received timely and standardized treatment and prevented concealment and omission of cases (Table 4).

5.4 Vector control

During the annual malaria transmission season, some natural villages that carried out fMDA also implemented control measures for Anopheles sinensis, the vector that transmits malaria, including indoor spraying of insecticides and the use of insecticide-treated mosquito nets. For example, in Huaibei City in 2007, villages with a high incidence of malaria soaked more than 1200 mosquito nets in insecticide and implemented large-scale spraying of 100,000 square meters with pesticides. At the same time, the villages also received comprehensive prevention and control measures such as vigorous environmental management and removal of mosquito breeding sites. Table 5 shows the number of people receiving fMDA and the number of

Table 4 Diagnosis of types of vivax malaria cases reported in Anhui Province from 2004 to 2015.

Year	Total	Clinically diagnosed cases	Confirmed cases	Suspected cases
2005	15,786	4241	11,469	76
2006	35,165	15,096	19,920	149
2007	27,509	8970	18,448	91
2008	13,537	3656	9855	26
2009	5231	1416	3796	19
2010	1451	519	930	2
2011	552	233	318	1
2012	41	1	40	0
2013	35	0	35	0
2014	27	0	27	0
2015	36	0	36	0
Total	99,370	34,132	64,874	364

Table 5 Implementation of treatment measures for malaria epidemic sites in Anhui Province from 2007 to 2015.

	Number of people taking fMDA		Number of people protected by insecticides	
Year	Before the start of transmission season	During the transmission season	Indoor spray	Medicated mosquito nets
2007	129,424	1,716,760	140,000	5027
2008	1,762,991	10,470	98,800	0
2009	968,059	9600	102,108	0
2010	703,006	25,865	119,430	5
2011	370,794	739	29,334	200
2012	193,355	2316	7313	0
2013	44,650	539	3289	1296
2014	12,582	314	912	334
2015	506	145	1094	207

people protected by pesticides in the province from 2007 to 2015. It can be seen from the table that in the disposal of malaria epidemic sites in Anhui Province, vector control measures are auxiliary measures of fMDA.

6. Effectiveness of the response to the resurgence

6.1 Malaria situation after taking medicine

After MDA implementation in the key populations, the malaria burden in the province declined rapidly, and the reported incidence rate dropped from 57.2/100,000 in 2006 to no local malaria cases since 2014.

In 2007, three rounds of fMDA of piperaquine phosphate curbed the trend of increasing incidence for 7 consecutive years. In the first half of 2007, the number of malaria cases in the province increased by 156.03% compared with the same period in 2006 but decreased by 21.95% over the course of the year compared with 2006 (Fig. 12).

In 2008 and 2009, the number of malaria cases in the province dropped by 50.69% and 56.23%, respectively, compared with the previous year. Until 2014, there was no local infection of vivax malaria in the province (Fig. 13), and the transmission area was shrinking year by year (Fig. 14) (Xu et al., 2015). Correspondingly, the composition ratio of Anhui cases

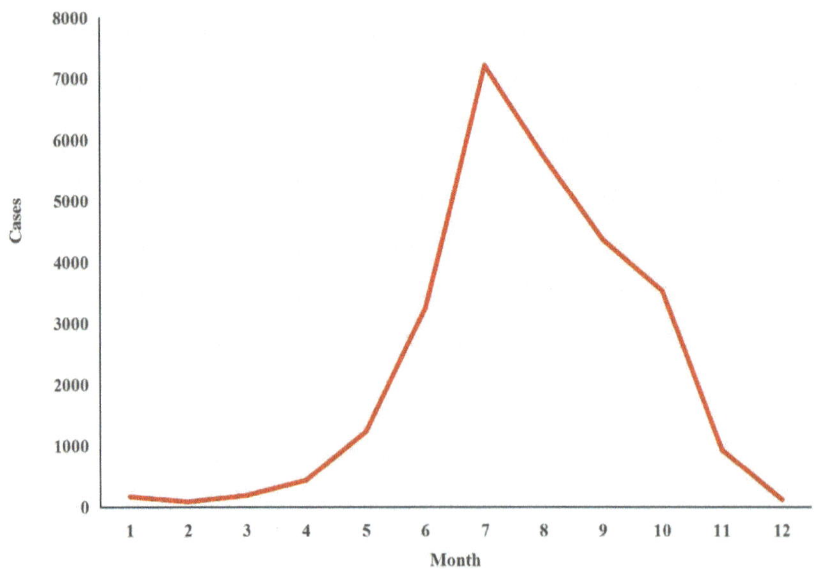

Fig. 12 Number of malaria cases in Anhui Province in 2007.

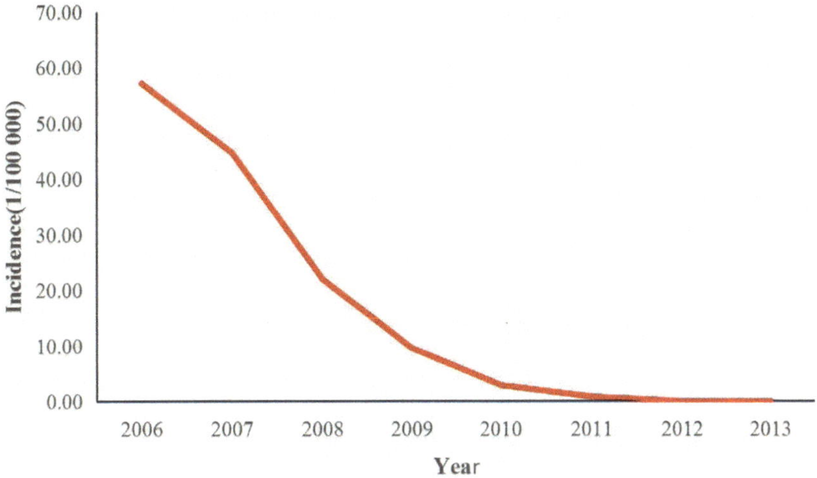

Fig. 13 The incidence of malaria in Anhui Province from 2006 to 2013

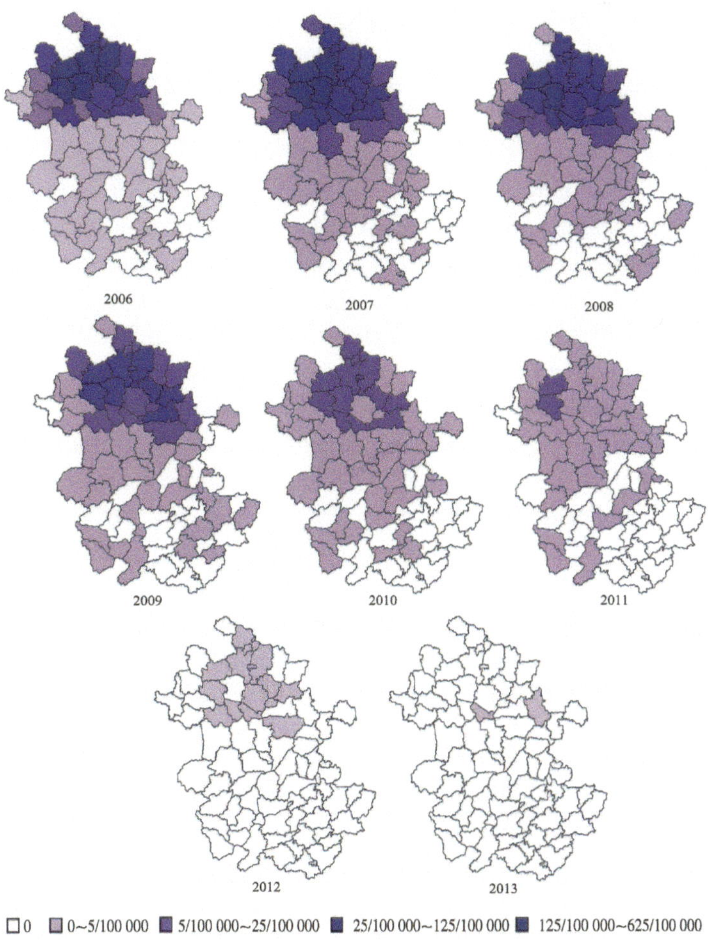

Fig. 14 The distribution of indigenous malaria with different incidences at the county level in Anhui Province during 2006–2013 (Xu, et al., 2015).

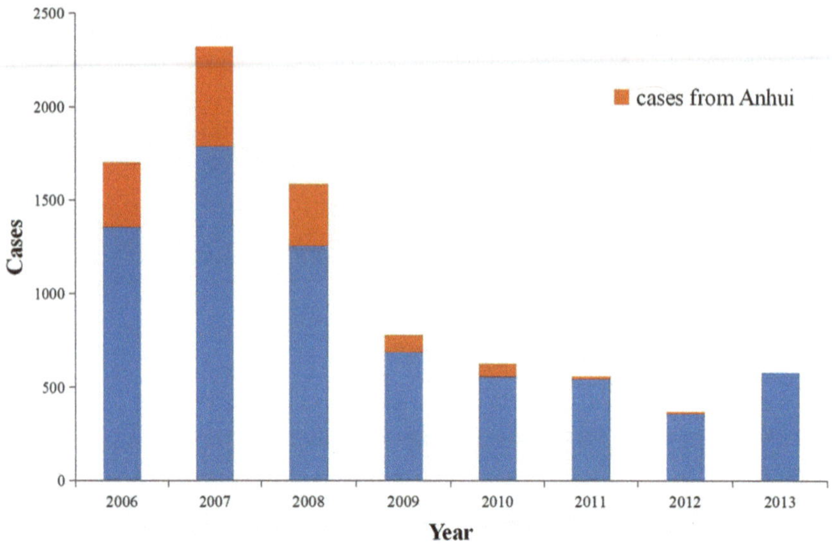

Fig. 15 Number of malaria cases, including those from Anhui in Shanghai, Zhejiang and Jiangsu Provinces, from 2006 to 2013.

in Shanghai, Zhejiang, and Jiangsu, the main labour exporting provinces of Anhui Province, also dropped from 25% in 2006 to 0 in 2013 (Fig. 15). MDA implementation has played a key role in the decline of *P. vivax* malaria in Anhui Province and even in central and eastern China, laying a solid foundation for China to achieve malaria elimination in 2021.

Unlike the clear effect in the control of vivax malaria, the role of MDA in the control of falciparum malaria was once questioned and was considered a historic failure. Because the implementation of MDA requires strong logistical support, there are ethical problems for some countries, and there is a risk of inducing drug resistance, resulting in a low rate of compliance (Finn et al., 2020a,b). Studies have shown that these earlier MDAs have a short implementation time, low coverage and poor compliance and lack the support of other interventions, such as good vector control and high-quality case management. Moreover, poor compliance and monotherapy may lead to drug resistance (Finn et al., 2020a,b).

6.2 Malaria diagnosis competency deficiency

In some places, not all malaria cases have been discovered. On the one hand, doctors have low diagnostic competency and miss diagnoses of cases with atypical symptoms. It could also be due to insufficient understanding of the symptoms, or malaria microscopy failed to detect the infection due to insufficient staining time or unstandardized dye solution. It is also possible that some cases were diagnosed but not registered, detailed investigations were not carried out before the implementation of MDA, and the list of malaria cases held by local medical institutions was not obtained. Therefore, doctors omitted some confirmed cases, clinically diagnosed cases, suspected cases, and asymptomatic cases, thereby reducing the area targeted by MDA.

7. Conclusions and perspectives

7.1 Conclusions

This article summarizes the background, specific conditions, main measures, steps and effects of the implementation of MDA to achieve control of the local *P. vivax* malaria epidemic in Anhui Province, located in Huanghuai Plain of central China. It was found that fMDA is feasible, effective and sustainable for the control of *P. vivax* malaria epidemics in temperate zones. There are some lessons learned that need to be emphasized: (i) the medication coverage area needs to be determined according to the characteristics of the malaria parasitic strain. Since malaria parasites have a long incubation period in this province, intrahepatic-phase parasite infection is mainly considered when delimiting the scope of medication coverage. The basic factors influencing the delineation of coverage areas are the number of malaria cases and bodies of water where mosquitos have bred in the previous 3 years; this is a more scientific approach than the previous selection of subjects based on malaria morbidity alone. However, the applicability of this approach to other countries and regions needs to be further studied; (ii) the proper drugs need to be selected according to the antimalarial mechanism of the drug and its half-life in the body, and it is important to identify the appropriate time to administer drugs according to the time of malaria transmission. There are certain times of the day that are better for drug delivery and observation of adverse drug reactions; (iii) the DOT method ensures coverage, compliance and the safety of the medication, and choosing the right person to deliver medicine can increase compliance; (iv) government leadership, extensive community participation and promotion of a positive atmosphere are necessary conditions for the implementation of MDA; (v) adequately preparing for the deployment of drugs and materials, obtaining informed consent and cooperation, observing the occurrence of adverse reactions, addressing adverse reactions, managing drugs strictly and collecting basic data and an overview of all malaria cases are also indispensable factors behind the success of a program.

7.2 Perspectives

Due to the implementation of measures focused on controlling the source of infection, the *P. vivax* malaria resurgence has been effectively controlled in Anhui Province. To strengthen the effects of prevention and control, prevention and control strategies have gradually changed from "targeting high-incidence areas and reducing the incidence" to "targeting each focus and eliminating infections". When the incidence rate in the previous 3 years was greater than or equal to 1/10000, the focus shifted to increasing medication dispersal and standardizing the treatment of patients during the non-peak period. When the incidence rate was less than 1/10000 in the previous 3 years, the focus shifted to epidemic surveillance, epidemiological investigation, and disease spot-treatment. Finally, when there were no local infection cases for three consecutive years, the focus shifted to improving the sensitivity of case monitoring and strengthening capacity building. Therefore, we put forward the following recommendations.

First, attention should be given to the coverage area of MDA or fMDA. Since MDA cannot achieve 100% coverage of the population in a given area during the implementation process and some highly mobile people cannot be reached during implementation, multiple rounds of MDA have been missed (Finn et al., 2020a,b). There are also those who refuse to take medication and have drug contraindications; therefore, some surviving cases or carriers can reinjection malaria parasites back into the community (Finn et al., 2020a,b). If these individuals are not diagnosed and treated in time, the spread of malaria may resume and eventually reach the previous morbidity and epidemic levels. Thus, MDA will only have a short-term effect in reducing the prevalence and morbidity of malaria (Eisele et al., 2020). The results from Zambia show that only high coverage of continuous mosquito vector control, good case management and improved surveillance systems can produce the desired results long-term; after the last round of MDA campaigns, the prevalence rate will drop to <1% for 15 months.

Second, it is better to integrate MDA with other measures to ensure that the expected results are achieved. Maintaining the incidence of malaria below 1% is very important for the malaria elimination plan. The establishment of a comprehensive case-based surveillance system is a prerequisite for malaria elimination (Eisele et al., 2020). Therefore, since the implementation of MDA is time-limited, after MDA, it is necessary to maintain high coverage of effective mosquito control, good case management, and a strong surveillance system (Daniels et al., 2020). If MDA is to be implemented, the effective implementation of other interventions, such as case diagnosis and treatment, effective mosquito vector control and other measures must be maintained. If combined with effective vector control with a high level of coverage and access management of good cases, the effect can be maintained for a long time after the MDA ceases (Brady et al., 2017). These core interventions can not only maximize the effect of MDA in controlling the epidemic but also maintain the effect after the intervention ceases.

Third, the surveillance and response systems must be guided and sustained even in the post-transmission period. In controlling the vivax malaria epidemic, the effectiveness of MDA depends on high coverage. At the same time, MDA is only one of the comprehensive prevention and control measures for the control and elimination of malaria in China. The significance of this method for achieving these goals cannot be accurately measured. Therefore, for the goal of malaria elimination, MDA needs to be implemented on a large scale with high-quality vector control. In addition, it is also necessary to establish an effective case monitoring response system based on diagnostic and treatment services to maintain the effectiveness of MDA (Eisele et al., 2020), thereby accelerating the elimination of malaria and preventing imported cases of malaria from spreading.

Last but not least, malaria elimination in China is not the final goal. We have to further strengthen the established surveillance and response systems at all levels to prevent malaria resurgence as well as small outbreaks in the high-risk areas where the mobile population is dominant.

Acknowledgements

We thank Prof Xiao-Nong Zhou and Dr. Jian-Hai Yin from National Institute of Parasitic Diseases, Chinese Center for Disease Control and Prevention for their revisions and suggestions on this article, and Dr. Yan-Song Bo from Huaibei City Center for Disease Control and Prevention, Dr. Feng Liu from Yongqiao County Center for Disease Control and Prevention, Dr. Pei-JunWang from Dingyuan County Center for Disease Control and Prevention for their supporting materials. And this review was supported in part by the Bill & Melinda Gates Foundation (No. INV-018913).

References

ACCESS-SMC Partnership, 2020. Effectiveness of seasonal malaria chemoprevention at scale in west and central Africa: an observational study. Lancet 396, 1829–1840. https://doi.org/10.1016/S0140-6736(20)32227-3. PMID: 33278936; PMCID: PMC7718580.

Anhui Provincial Department of Health, 2007. Implementation Plan for The Elimination of Malaria Infection Sources in Anhui Province in 2007.

Anhui Provincial Department of Health, 2010. Implementation Plan for The Malaria Rest Period Medication in Anhui Province in 2010.

Baba, E., Hamade, P., Kivumbi, H., Marasciulo, M., Maxwell, K., Moroso, D., Roca-Feltrer, A., Sanogo, A., Stenstrom, J.J., Tibenderana, J., Abdoulaye, R., Coulibaly, P., Hubbard, E., Jah, H., Lama, E.K., Razafindralambo, L., Van Hulle, S., Jagoe, G., Tchouatieu, A.-M., Collins, D., Gilmartin, C., Tetteh, G., Djibo, Y., Ndiaye, F., Kalleh, M., Kandeh, B., Audu, B., Ntadom, G., Kiba, A., Savodogo, Y., Boulotigam, K., Sougoudi, D.A., Guilavogui, T., Keita, M., Kone, D., Jackou, H., Ouba, I., Ouedraogo, E., Messan, H.A., Jah, F., Kaira, M.J., Sano, M.S., Traore, M.C., Ngarnaye, N., Elagbaje, A.Y.C., Halleux, C., Merle, C., Iessa, N., Pal, S., Sefiani, H., Souleymani, R., Laminou, I., Doumagoum, D., Kesseley, H., Coldiron, M., Grais, R., Kana, M., Ouedraogo, J.B., Zongo, I., Eloike, T., Ogboi, S.J., Achan, J., Bojang, K., Ceesay, S., Dicko, A., Djimde, A., Sagara, I., Diallo, A., NdDiaye, J.L., Loua, K.M., Beshir, K., Cairns, M., Fernandez, Y., Lal, S., Mansukhani, R., Muwanguzi, J., Scott, S., Snell, P., Sutherland, C., Tuta, R., Milligan, P., 2020. Effectiveness of seasonal malaria chemoprevention at scale in west and central africa: an observational study. Lancet 396, 1829–1840.

Bennett, A., Porter, T.R., Mwenda, M.C., Yukich, J.O., Finn, T.P., Lungu, C., Silumbe, K., Mambwe, B., Chishimba, S., Mulube, C., Bridges, D.J., Hamainza, B., Slutsker, L., Steketee, R.W., Miller, J.M., Eisele, T.P., 2020. A longitudinal cohort to monitor malaria infection incidence during mass drug administration in Southern Province, Zambia. Am. J. Trop. Med. Hyg. 103 (2_Suppl), 54–65. https://doi.org/10.4269/ajtmh.19-0657. PMID: 32618245; PMCID: PMC7416973.

Brady, O.J., Slater, H.C., Pemberton-Ross, P., Wenger, E., Maude, R.J., Ghani, A.C., Penny, M.A., Gerardin, J., White, L.J., Chitnis, N., Aguas, R., Hay, S.I., Smith, D.L., Stuckey, E.M., Okiro, E.A., Smith, T.A., Okell, L.C., 2017. Role of mass drug administration in elimination of plasmodium falciparum malaria: a consensus modelling study. Lancet Glob. Health 5, e680–e687.

Chen, J., Liu, W.F., 2021. Anhui Statistical Yearbook-2021. China Statistics Press. http://tjj.ah.gov.cn/oldfiles/tjj/tjjweb/tjnj/2021/cn.html.

Cheng, J.S., Wang, J.J., Xu, X., 2013. Investigation on relationship between malaria incidence and migrant history of migrant farmer workers and their family members in Bozhou City. Chin. J. Dis. Control. Prev. 17 (1), 45–47.

Daniels, R.F., Schaffner, S.F., Bennett, A., Porter, T.R., Yukich, J.O., Mulube, C., Mambwe, B., Mwenda, M.C., Chishimba, S., Bridges, D.J., Moonga, H., Hamainza, B., ChizemaKawesha, E., Miller, J.M., Steketee, R.W., Wirth, D.F., Eisele, T.P., Hartl, D.L., Volkman, S.K., 2020. Evidence for reduced malaria parasite population after application of population-level antimalarial drug strategies in southern province, zambia. Am. J. Trop. Med. Hyg. 103 (2_Suppl), 66–73.

Deng, C., Huang, B., Wang, Q., Wu, W., Zheng, S., Zhang, H., Li, D., Feng, D., Li, G., Xue, L., Yang, T., Tuo, F., Mohadji, F., Su, X.Z., Xu, Q., Wu, Z., Lin, L., Zhou, J., Yan, H., Bacar, A., Said, A.K., Keke, R.A., MsaMliva, A., Mohamed, M., Wang, X., Huang, S., Oithik, F., Li, X.B., Lu, F., Fay, M.P., Liu, X.H., Wellems, T.E., Song, J., 2018. Large-scale artemisinin-piperaquine mass drug administration with or without primaquine dramatically reduces malaria in a highly endemic region of Africa. Clin. Infect. Dis. 67, 1670–1676.

Eisele, T.P., Bennett, A., Silumbe, K., Finn, T.P., Porter, T.R., Chalwe, V., Hamainza, B., Moonga, H., Kooma, E., ChizemaKawesha, E., Kamuliwo, M., Yukich, J.O., Keating, J., Schneider, K., Conner, R.O., Earle, D., Slutsker, L., Steketee, R.W., Miller, J.M., 2020. Impact of four rounds of mass drug administration with dihydroartemisinin-piperaquine implemented in Southern Province, Zambia. Am. J. Trop. Med. Hyg. 103 (2_Suppl), 7–18.

Fehr, A., Nieto-Sanchez, C., Muela, J., Jaiteh, F., Ceesay, O., Maneh, E., Baldeh, D., Achan, J., Dabira, E., Conteh, B., Bunders-Aelen, J., Smekens, T., Broekhuizen, H., D'Alessandro, U., Peeters Grietens, K., 2021. From informed consent to adherence: factors influencing involvement in mass drug administration with ivermectin for malaria elimination in the Gambia. Malar. J. 20 (1), 198.

Finn, T.P., Porter, T.R., Moonga, H., Silumbe, K., Daniels, R.F., Volkman, S.K., Yukich, J.O., Keating, J., Bennett, A., Steketee, R.W., Miller, J.M., Eisele, T.P., 2020a. Adherence to mass drug administration with dihydroartemisinin-piperaquine and plasmodium falciparum clearance in Southern Province, Zambia. Am. J. Trop. Med. Hyg. 103 (2_Suppl), 37–45.

Finn, T.P., Yukich, J.O., Bennett, A., Porter, T.R., Lungu, C., Hamainza, B., ChizemaKawesha, E., Conner, R.O., Silumbe, K., Steketee, R.W., Miller, J.M., Keating, J., Eisele, T.P., 2020b. Treatment coverage estimation for mass drug administration for malaria with dihydroartemisinin-piperaquine in Southern Province, Zambia. Am. J. Trop. Med. Hyg. 103 (2_Suppl), 19–27.

Gou, J.B., Feng, Z.J., Li, H.Z., Zheng, C.J., Ge, J., Zhu, G., You, F.H., Zhu, D.S., 2008. Analysis of side effects caused by piperaquinephosphate for malaria prophylaxis in population. China Trop. Med. 4, 541–543.

Hsiang, M.S., Hwang, J., Tao, A.R., Liu, Y., Bennett, A., Shanks, G.D., Cao, J., Kachur, S.P., Feachem, R.G., Gosling, R.D., Gao, Q., 2013. Mass drug administration for the control and elimination of plasmodium vivax malaria: an ecological study from Jiangsu province. China. Malar J. 12, 383.

Jiang, J.J., Zhang, T., Xu, X., Lü, X.F., Wang, S.Q., Tian, C.C., Li, W.D., 2020. Surveillance of malaria vectors in Anhui province from 2016 to 2018. Chin. J. Schistosomiasis Control 32, 389–392.

Keys, H., Urena, K., Reyes, J., Bardosh, K., Pell, C., Puello, J., Blount, S., Noland, G.S., 2021. Rapid ethnographic assessment for potential antimalarial mass drug administration in an outbreak area of Santo Domingo, Dominican Republic. Malar. J. 20, 76.

Liu, Y.X., 2007. Study of geographic information system on the incidence of malaria in Anhui. J. Dis. Cont. 11, 379–382.

Liu, H., Xu, J.W., Bi, Y., 2018. Malaria burden and treatment targets in Kachin special region ii, Myanmar from 2008 to 2016: a retrospective analysis. PLoS One 13, e0195032.

Murta, F.L.G., Marques, L.L.G., Santos, A.P.C., Batista, T.S.B., Mendes, M.O., Silva, E.D., Neto, A.V.S., Fabiano, M., Rodovalho, S.R., Monteiro, W.M., MVG, L., 2021. Perceptions about malaria among Brazilian gold miners in an Amazonian border area: perspectives for malaria elimination strategies. Malar. J. 20, 286. https://doi.org/10.1186/s12936-021-03820-0. PMID: 34174880; PMCID: PMC8236171.

Nadia, J., Lu, F., 2022. Historical experiences on mass drug administration for malaria control and elimination, its challenges and China's experience: a narrative review. Acta Trop., 106209. https://doi.org/10.1016/j.actatropica.2021.106209.

Pan, B., 2003. Morphological characteristics, ecological features and the role in malaria transmission of the major malaria transmission vectors in China. J. Trop. Med. 3, 477–480.

Shen, Y.Z., 2006. Investigation on transmission factors of malaria in Anopheles sinensis areas in Anhui Province. J. Pathog. Biol. 04, 301–303.

Shen, Y.Z., Zou, Z., Lu, H.X., Chen, J.M., Li, H.M., 1998. Prevention and control measures and effect evaluation of falciparum malaria in Anhui Province. Anhui J. Prev. Med. 02, 75–77.

Silumbe, K., Finn, T.P., Jennings, T., Sikombe, C., Chiyende, E., Hamainza, B., ChizemaKawesha, E., Eisele, T.P., Earle, D., Steketee, R.W., Miller, J.M., 2020. Assessment of the acceptability of testing and treatment during a mass drug administration trial for malaria in Zambia using mixed methods. Am. J. Trop. Med. Hyg. 103 (2_Suppl), 28–36.

Wang, J.J., Li, W.D., Shen, Y.Z., Xu, X., Jiang, J.J., 2006. Technical Report of China/WHO 2006 Annual Cooperation Project "Study of Malaria Transmission Characteristics in Anhui Province". WP/2006/CHN/MAL/1.2/001.

Wang, J.J., Li, W.D., Shen, Y.Z., Xu, X., Jiang, J.J., 2009. Technical Report of China/WHO 2008/2009 Annual Cooperation Project "Discussion on Malaria Control Mode in Anopheles Sinensis Area of Anhui Province". WP/2008/CHN/02 02.02.

World Health Organization, 2021. World Malaria Report 2021. WHO, Geneva.

Xia, Z.G., Xu, J.F., Zhang, S.S., Wang, R.B., Qian, Y.J., Zhou, S.S., Yang, W.Z., Zhou, X.N., 2014. Determination of key interventions for the transition from control to felimiantion of malaria in China. Chin J. Schisto. Control 6, 598–601.

Xu, F.N., Shen, Y.Z., Jia, S.C., Zou, Z., 2003. Feature analysis of local malaria re-rise in plasmodium vivax endemic area in ANHUI Province. J. Pathog. Biol. 01, 23–25.

Xu, B.L., Su, Y.P., Liu, Y., 2011. Malaria evaluation on the control effect in Henan Province during 1970–2010. Henan J. Prev. Med. 22, 321–326.

Xu, X., Li, W.D., Jiang, J.J., Zhang, T., Wang, J.J., 2015. Analysis of malaria epidemic characteristics in Anhui province during 1999–2013. Chin. J. Parasitol. Parasitic Dis. 33, 1–6.

Xu, J.W., Li, J.J., Guo, H.P., Pu, S.W., Li, S.M., Wang, R.H., Liu, H., Wang, W.J., 2017. Malaria from hyperendemicity to elimination in Hekou County on China-Vietnam border: an ecological study. Malar. J. 16, 66. https://doi.org/10.1186/s12936-017-1709-z. PMID: 28173802; PMCID: PMC5297092.

Xu, X., Zhang, T., Jiang, J.J., Li, W.D., 2020. Course of malaria control and elimination in Anhui Province. J. Trop. Dis. Parasitol. 18, 65–69. 80.

Yuan, Y.C., Wu, Z.Y., Kan, S.P., Li, Q.B., Chen, F.Q., Wu, F.L., Lou, Y.S., Huang, Q.L., Shen, Y.Z., Zhu, H.P., Zou, Z., Li, Y.Q., Fan, H.J., Chen, J.M., Xuan, S.Z., 1990. Research on the transmission vector of falciparum malaria in Anhui. Anhui Med. J. 04, 48–50.

Yuan, Y.C., Wu, Z.Y., Li, Q.B., Wu, F.L., Kan, S.P., 1991. Distribution of Anopheles anthropophagus and its role in spreading malaria and filariasis in Anhui Province. J. Pathog. Biol. 01, 58–60.

Zhao, X., Thanapongtharm, W., Lawawirojwong, S., Wei, C., Tang, Y., Zhou, Y., Sun, X., Sattabongkot, J., Kaewkungwal, J., 2020. Spatiotemporal trends of malaria in relation to economic development and cross-border movement along the China-Myanmar border in Yunnan Province. Korean J. Parasitol. 58, 267–278. https://doi.org/10.3347/kjp.2020.58.3.267. Epub 2020 Jun 26. PMID: 32615740; PMCID: PMC7338897.

Zhou, S.S., Wang, Y., Tang, L.H., 2007. National malaria situation in 2006. Chin. J. Parasitol. Parasitic Dis. 25, 439–441.

Zhu, D.S., Yang, W.Z., Li, H.Z., Zheng, C.J., Gou, J.B., 2007. Analysis of characteristics of malaria incidence and measures for treatment of malaria in the periods of inactivity in the unstable areas of central China. China Trop. Med. 7, 1281–1284.

Zhu, A.Y., Xu, J.J., Geng, Y., Li, A.M., Lin, G.C., 2011. Evaluation of therapeutic measures of radical treatment for malaria in pre-transmission season in four key counties of malaria control of Guizhou in 2009. Modern Prev. Med. 22, 4749–4750. 4756.

Zhu, D.S., Wang, J.J., Xu, X., Zhu, J., Li, H.Z., 2013. Evaluating the effect of preventive medicine for residents living around mosquito breeding water during rest period of malaria. Chin. J. Prev. Med. 1, 44–47.

Zou, Z., Lu, H.X., Shen, Y.Z., Chen, J.M., Wu, Z.Y., Xu, F.N., 2000. Research on the prevalence and prevention of falciparum malaria in Anhui Province. J. Dis. Cont. 4, 307.

CHAPTER FIVE

One Health approach to improve the malaria elimination programme in Henan Province

Ying Liu[a], Zhi-Quan He[a], Dan Wang[a], Ya-Bo Hu[b], Dan Qian[a], Cheng-Yun Yang[a], Rui-min Zhou[a], Su-Hua Li[a], De-Ling Lu[a], and Hong-Wei Zhang[a,*]

[a]Henan Center for Disease Control and Prevention, Zhengzhou, Henan, PR China
[b]Zhengzhou University, Zhengzhou, Henan, PR China
*Corresponding author: e-mail address: zhwei69@163.com

Contents

1. Introduction 155
   1.1 Phase in control of epidemics (1950–1979) 155
   1.2 Phase of primary malaria elimination (1980–1994) 156
   1.3 Phase of consolidating the control achievements (1995–2009) 156
   1.4 Phase of malaria elimination (since 2010) 158
2. One Health approach applied in malaria control programme 159
   2.1 Concept development of One Health 159
   2.2 One Health approach applied in malaria control programme 159
3. The elimination of malaria with One Health approach in Henan Province 160
   3.1 The working principle of government-led and departmental collaboration (multi-sectoral cooperation) 160
   3.2 Multi-provincial cooperation 161
   3.3 Integrated strategies to eliminate infectious sources combined with vector control (multidisciplinary cooperation) 163
4. Case studies on implementation of One Health approach in malaria control in Henan Province 166
   4.1 Response to malaria re-emergence in Yongcheng county 166
   4.2 The conversion of dry land to lotus ponds stimulated malaria outbreak 168
   4.3 Outbreak of *Falciparum* malaria from migrant population in Taikang county 168
5. Introduction of malaria control technologies supported by One Health approach 170
   5.1 Genetic tracking of *Vivax* malaria 170
   5.2 Bacterial larvicides for malaria control in Yongcheng county 170

Advances in Parasitology, Volume 116
ISSN 0065-308X
https://doi.org/10.1016/bs.apar.2022.02.001

6. One Health approach applied in prevention of malaria retransmission 171
6.1 Surveillance of imported cases 171
6.2 Management of imported cases 172
6.3 Treatment of imported cases 173
6.4 Reference laboratory network 174
6.5 Entomological surveillance and vector control 176
6.6 Public health education and health promotion 177
6.7 Research on socio-economic factors 179
7. Lessons learnt from malaria control and elimination in Henan Province 179
7.1 Attentions of governments at all levels were paid, which provided organizational foundation and facilitated the actions on malaria elimination 179
7.2 Efficient mechanism of multi-regional joint control promoted malaria elimination in grand regions at large 180
7.3 Comprehensive control measures acted as an important role in malaria control 180
7.4 Scientific researches on this field provided strong support to malaria elimination 181
7.5 Risks for re-establishment of malaria 181
8. Conclusions and perspectives 182
8.1 Conclusions 182
8.2 Perspectives 182
Acknowledgements 183
References 183

Abstract

One Health is a collaborative, multi-sectoral, trans-disciplinary approach with the goal of achieving optimal health outcomes by recognizing the interconnection between people, animals, plants, and the environment and determining how this relates to the control of infectious diseases such as malaria, schistosomiasis and so on. Malarias caused by *Plasmodium* that commonly infects female *Anopheles* mosquitoes, which feed on human blood and act as a disease vector. It has been a worldwide important public health problem from ancient times. Also, malaria is one of the infectious diseases with the longest epidemic time and the most serious harm in the history of Henan Province, China. During the past decades, the multi-sectoral, cross-regional, and multi-disciplinary One Health approach contributed to a significant reduction in malaria incidence, resulting in initiation of the Henan Malaria Elimination Action Plan. Herein, we reviewed the history of the fight against malaria in Henan Province. A full picture of malaria epidemics, prevention, and control strategies were showed, with the objective that it will help stakeholders, and policy-makers to take informed decisions on public health issues and intervention designs on malaria control towards elimination in the similar areas.

1. Introduction

Henan Province, located in the Middle-lower Yellow River, east-central of China and borders with Anhui and Shandong to the east, Shanxi and Hebei to the north, Shaanxi to the west and Hubei to the south. Henan has a humid warm-temperate climate, with four distinct seasons: cold and dry in winter, hot and rainy in summer. The annual temperature is 12.7–16.2 °C, and the annual rainfall is 477.8–1167.3 mm. Henan Province was an endemic area of malaria historically (Zhang et al., 2006b). *Plasmodium vivax* (*P. vivax*) was distributed all over the province, while *Plasmodium falciparum* (*P. falciparum*) was endemic in the area south of 33°N before 1987, and *Plasmodium malariae* (*P. malariae*) was diffusely distributed in the area south of 33°N in the 1950s (Shang et al., 2011). *Anopheles sinensis* (*An. sinensis*) and *Anopheles anthropophagus* (*An. anthropophagus*) are the main malaria vectors. *An. sinensis* can be found throughout the province, and is the dominant species of the genus *Anopheles* in Henan Province, while *An. anthropophagus* was the main transmission vector of *falciparum* malaria and distributed in 10 counties south of 33° N, which was consistent with the epidemic areas of *P. falciparum*. In Henan, malaria control and elimination programme can be divided into four phases: control of epidemics, basic malaria elimination, consolidating control achievements, and malaria elimination (Zhang et al., 2019).

1.1 Phase in control of epidemics (1950–1979)

At this stage, all the malaria-endemic areas established institutions for the prevention and control of malaria. These institutions put forward comprehensive prevention and control strategies that focused on controlling the source of infection under the plan named "two treatment, one prevention, extensive vector control," which means treatment of patients with malaria, radical treatment in spring, drug prophylaxis in the transmission season and vector control activities. A total of 38,292,000 patients with malaria were treated, 171,214,000 residents were cured in the resting phase, and 253,698,000 residents took medicine against malaria in the transmission season. By 1979, the incidence had decreased to 0.58%, representing a decline by 96.00% relative to that in 1970, and more than 5% of the counties hadn't detected newly infected cases in Henan Province.

1.2 Phase of primary malaria elimination (1980–1994)

During the primary elimination phase, the malaria control strategy of the entire province was adjusted as follows: Comprehensive measures that paid equal attention to the control of the *Anopheles* vector and management of the source of infection were used in malaria-endemic areas with *An. Anthropophagus*. A prevention and control strategy of improving malaria surveillance was adopted in areas where the incidence dropped below 1/10,000. In addition, blood tests for *plasmodium* were gradually conducted in febrile patients, and 21,849,000 patients with fever received microscopic examination of blood smears for *plasmodium* (microscopic examination). There is a significant reduction in malaria burden during this phase. The number of *falciparum* cases decreased rapidly, and there had been no indigenous *falciparum* patients since 1988, the elimination of *falciparum* malaria had been successfully achieved. By 1994, all counties had been confirmed through provincial assessment to meet the standard of basic malaria elimination promulgated by the Ministry of Health, that is, annual incidence of malaria below 1/10,000 for three consecutive years by county.

1.3 Phase of consolidating the control achievements (1995–2009)

The epidemic situation fluctuated at low levels in most malaria-endemic areas, with sporadic cases reported during this phase. However, due to various reasons, epidemics rebounded and broke out locally in the Huanghuai plain covering eastern Henan and mid-north Anhui. In 2006, Henan Province successively launched contingency plans for malaria emergency response at outbreak areas, Yongcheng county, strengthened leadership and investment in malaria prevention and control, implemented improved measures including expanded radical treatment, early and effective case management, indoor residual sprays (IRS) and larviciding, thus effectively containing the continued increase trend in resurgence areas. In 2003–2010, with the support of the Global Fund to fight AIDS, Tuberculosis and Malaria (GFATM), the malaria control campaigns were performed successively in 2 counties (round 1, 2003–2008) and 15 counties (round 5, 2006–2010). The GFATM Project offered equipment, drugs, and other supplies for malaria control in addition to funding training and supporting intervention activities, paved the way to initiate the malaria elimination programme in 2010. By 2009, no cases had been reported in 89 (55.97%) counties among all 159 counties, and the incidence rate was more than 10/10,000 in only 3counties (Fig. 1).

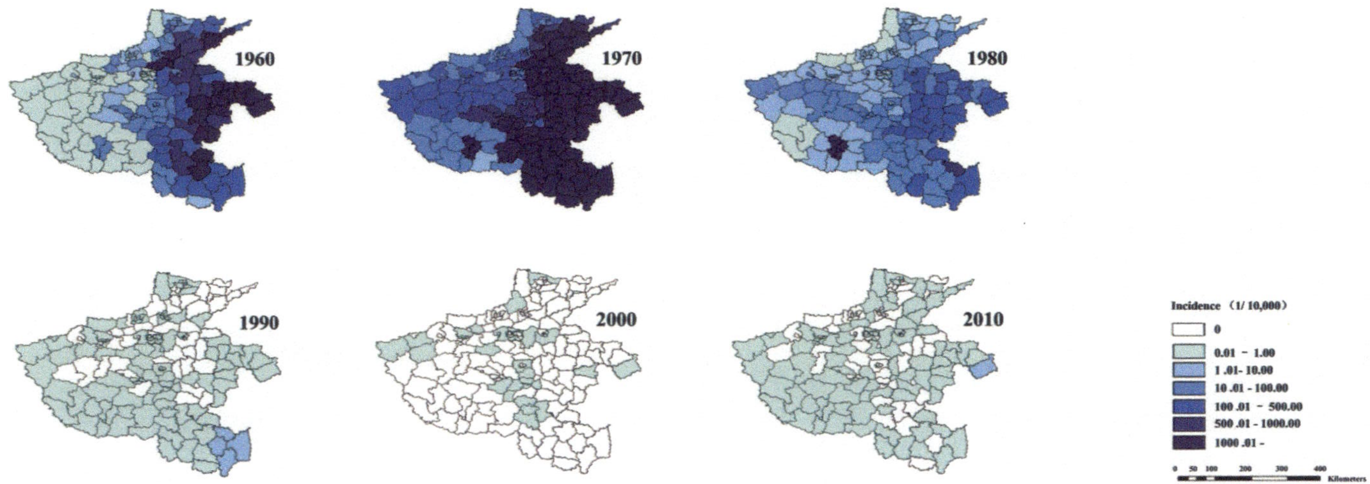

Fig. 1 The geographical stratification of malaria incidence based on the incidence in Henan Province (Guo et al., 2021).

1.4 Phase of malaria elimination (since 2010)

In 2010, the "Henan Province Malaria Elimination Action Plan (2010–2020)" was issued according to "China Malaria Elimination Action Plan (2010–2020)," with a goal of malaria elimination by 2018. The strategy of this phase was tracking malaria cases and response to clear each focus by following individual case. Moreover, 6 type I, 84 type II, and 69 type III malaria endemic counties were classified according to the national plan. Enhanced malaria control strategies and measures were taken in type 1 counties to further reduce the incidence. Malaria elimination strategies and measures were adopted in type 2 counties to achieve the goal of no indigenous cases as soon as possible. In type 3 counties, the monitoring and handling capability was further improved to prevent re-transmission due to imported cases. During this stage, malaria diagnosis network was established, the quality control system was improved, and malaria designated hospitals were set up. In 2012, no indigenous cases were reported for the first time, and all of 159 counties have passed verification for malaria-free by 2017. At present, about 200 malaria cases are diagnosed in Henan Province each year (Fig. 2) (Guo et al., 2021). Most of them were travellers and immigrants returning from malaria epidemic countries, especially from sub-Saharan Africa and Southeast Asia (Yang et al., 2021).

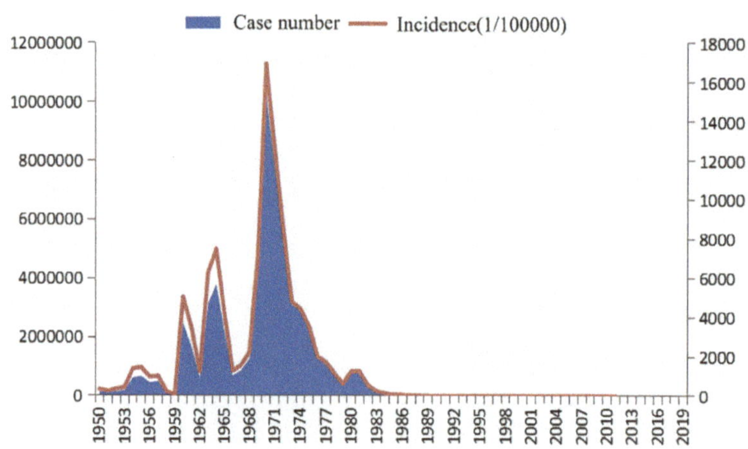

Fig. 2 Malaria epidemic situation in Henan Province, 1950–2019 (Guo et al., 2021).

2. One Health approach applied in malaria control programme

2.1 Concept development of One Health

The concept of One Health originated from One Medicine proposed by Schwabe in 1960 (Zinsstag et al., 2011). The One Health concept proposes a global expansion strategy for interdisciplinary collaboration and communication to improve the health of humans, animals, and the environment. This concept encourages public health professionals, clinicians, veterinarians, and other professionals from all areas to break down barriers between each other's disciplines to actively cooperate and communicate to explore new research across disciplines and regions. This collaborative, multidisciplinary framework is suggested to better address important issues such as emerging infectious diseases and environmental changes (Nie et al., 2016). Based on a systematic approach and multidisciplinary cooperation, the One Health strategy is an internationally recognized effective approach to managing emerging infectious diseases. It emphasizes the collective health of people, animals, and the environment, and promotes the prevention and control of emerging zoonotic infectious diseases by strengthening health monitoring of animals, occupationally exposed people, and the environment, which is the most cost-effective (Li et al., 2018).

2.2 One Health approach applied in malaria control programme

Malaria, a serious and sometimes fatal disease caused by *Plasmodium*, a parasite that commonly infects female *Anopheles* mosquitoes which feed on human blood, thus serving as a disease vector. Malaria is a great drain on many national economies and a public health problem worldwide. After arduous efforts for decades, the overall disease burden has been greatly reduced, and many countries have reached the standard of malaria elimination (WHO, 2021). However, the epidemic factors affecting malaria are complex, including both natural and social factors. Challenges remain in eradication malaria, including the resistance of mosquitoes to insecticides used to kill them, drug-resistant malaria parasites, and administrative issues (Sougoufara et al., 2017). Thus, malaria still remains high on the list of diseases that causes major health burdens, globally. At present, malaria is a complex public health problem that cannot be resolved by a single discipline, nor can a single institution or country resolve it. To effectively address the ongoing malaria crisis, the global population should pool their resources and expertise and break down disciplinary boundaries to use integrative approaches, taking the One Health concept as guidance. Although "One Health" is a relatively new term, this concept has existed for a long time (Zhou, 2021). Reviewing the history of malaria prevention and control efforts in Henan Province, multi-department cooperation, regional joint prevention and control strategies, and comprehensive prevention and control measures focusing on the source of infection precisely reflected the concept of the One Health approach (Aguirre et al., 2019).

3. The elimination of malaria with One Health approach in Henan Province

3.1 The working principle of government-led and departmental collaboration (multi-sectoral cooperation)

Henan's malaria prevention and control involves many departments under the unified leadership of governments at all levels. These departments include Health Commission, Customs, Education, Development and Reform Commission and Finance, and others, which cooperate closely to support all prevention and control measures. All levels of Center for Disease Control and Prevention (CDC) and medical institutions are specifically responsible for implementing malaria prevention and control through the three levels network of provincial, prefecture and county. In August 2010, the "Henan Province Malaria Elimination Action Plan (2010–2020)" was issued, which clearly established the goal and objective of the Malaria Elimination Campaign in Henan Province, as well as the responsibilities of relevant departments. Governments at all levels have integrated malaria elimination programme into the regional economic and social development plans and target management assessment content, and thus clarified the responsibilities and tasks of each department, strengthened the leadership, coordinated management, supervision and assessment, so as to ensure all the measures in place. The Provincial Health Commission is in charge of malaria elimination programme, and is responsible for formulating and organizing implementation of malaria elimination related policies, strategies and measures, and cooperating with relevant departments and establishing malaria expert groups on prevention and control and clinical treatment to provide intensive technical guidance. CDCs at all level are responsible for carrying out the activities of malaria elimination. Medical institutions at all levels and of all types are responsible for diagnosing, reporting, treating, and collaborating with CDCs for malaria elimination. The Development and Reform Commission and the Financial Department at all levels are in charge of incorporating malaria prevention and control into the all levels of economic and social development plan, and arranging special funds for malaria elimination. The education sectors are responsible for the health promotion and education of malaria prevention knowledge in primary and secondary schools. The radio and television administrations are responsible for various forms of dissemination about malaria prevention and control knowledge. The science and technology departments are responsible for the scientific research and application of the technologies and products related to malaria prevention and elimination. Entry-exit inspection and quarantine, public security, tourism, commerce and other departments are responsible for malaria health education, case surveillance, and entry-exit management on diseases prevention and control for relevant entry-exit population, and timely communicate with health departments to share relevant information (Fig. 3).

3.2 Multi-provincial cooperation

The multi-provincial cooperation of malaria prevention mechanism in the five province of Jiangsu, Shandong, Henan, Anhui, and Hubei began in 1974 and was approved by the State Council (Kong et al., 2016). As the species of *Plasmodium* and *Anopheles* vector were the same among these provinces and the ecological environments were similar in the region (Zhang, 1995), these five provinces simultaneously implemented common control strategies including seasonal mass drug administration (MDA) and other vector control strategies. Mutual supervision and inspection were conducted once annually to promote cooperative works. From 1974 to 1979, microscopic examination for *Plasmodium* were gradually conducted in patients with fever, and 838,800 patients with fever received microscopic examination for *Plasmodium* (Tang and Gao, 2013a). In addition, a total of 27.39 million malaria patients were treated across the five provinces, nearly 416,88 million residents were treated in spring, and 603,41million persons took anti-malaria drugs during the transmission season. These treatment regimens controlled the epidemic effectively and reduced malaria burden by 86.05%, from 13.73 million cases in 1973 to 1.91 million cases in 1979 (Tang and Gao, 2013b). During the past 40 years, the multi-provincial cooperation mechanism has improved the overall effectiveness of malaria elimination efforts and promoted malaria elimination in participating provinces (Liu et al., 2008).

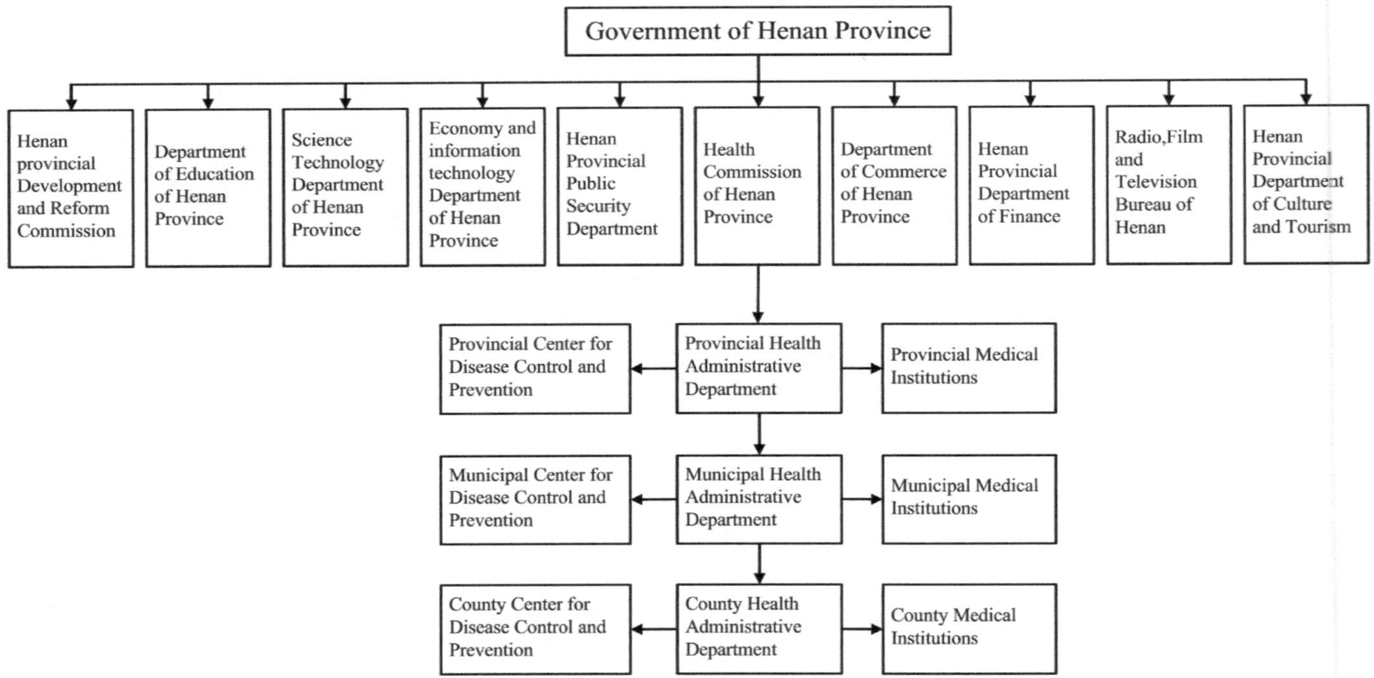

Fig. 3 Organization of malaria elimination in Henan Province.

3.3 Integrated strategies to eliminate infectious sources combined with vector control (multidisciplinary cooperation)

After primary elimination of malaria in Henan Province, malaria prevention and control strategies have been changed accordingly to avoid stagnation by maintaining the necessary investment in human, financial, and material resources. Comprehensive prevention and control measures have been implemented in areas where *An. sinensis* is the primary vector, focusing on timely detection and management of infection sources. In areas where *An. anthropophagus* is distributed, integrated measures for vector control and source management have been implemented. At the same time, all counties should detect and manage residual and imported cases in a timely manner to prevent outbreaks and consolidate the achievements.

3.3.1 Case detection

Case detection is a screening process in which the indicator is either the presence of fever or epidemiological attributes such as high-risk situations or groups. Cases can be detected by passive case detection or active case detection.

Passive case detection: The passive case detection refers as malaria cases among patients who visit health services for diagnosis and treatment health facility on their own initiative, usually for fever. From 1990 to 2005, a total of 11,216,100 patients with fever were tested for malaria, and the rate of microscopic examination was 0.06–2.06%. Among them, 11,213 patients tested positive, the positive rate was 0.01–0.81%, and the average positive rate was 0.10%. Therefore, 38,654 cases or suspected malaria cases were treated (Liu and Xu, 2006).

Active case detection: The active case detection refers to malaria screening for fever performed by health workers in communities and households, sometimes among population groups without fever who are considered at high risk. A total of 71,234 residents/primary school students were surveyed from 1993 to 1999, and 286 positive cases were found, with an average positive rate of 0.40%. In 1996, 2719 residents/primary school students were screened in 10 townships of 5 counties, including Pingqiao, Shihe, Gushi, Shangcheng and Tongbai, 117 *plasmodium*-positive cases were found, and the positive rate was 4.30%. The rates in Shihe and Tongbai were higher than other counties, 11.62% (43/370) and 15.94% (33/207), respectively. But when the year came to 2001, similar investigation was done in

Shihe county, 1080 residents/primary school students were investigated, and no positive cases were detected (Liu and Xu, 2006).

Serological monitoring: Sero-epidemiological studies usually be used to assess malaria transmission intensity (Voller and Bruce-Chwatt, 1968) and reductions in transmission (Cornille-Brögger et al., 1978). From 1990 to 2001, 34,846 people were tested with indirect fluorescence antibody test (IFAT), and 1149 were positive, the positive rate fluctuated from 0.80% to 13.05%. Between 2005 and 2010, the overall positive rate of IFAT was 4.16% (310/7453) in national surveillance sites in Henan Province (Liu et al., 2014b).

3.3.2 Radical treatment

P. vivax was the dominant parasite and distributed over the province. Detection of *P. vivax* is not easy because a large percentage of individuals in endemic areas can be asymptomatic and have submicroscopic blood levels of parasitemia (Baum et al., 2015). In addition, the WHO recommends a 14-day course of primaquine does not always clear *P. vivax* hypnozoites totally (Thriemer et al., 2017). Radical treatments, which were carried out before or at the start of a new malaria transmission season, can clear persistent liver-stage parasites effectively (Shang et al., 2006). Practice has proved that 180 mg primaquine for 8 days administered in spring is an appropriate way to eliminate the remaining infectious source, reduce relapse, and prevent the spread of malaria (Zhu et al., 2007). A variety of radical treatment regimens were administered through each stage of malaria control from hyperendemicity to elimination in the province. For example, to response the resurgence in Yongcheng county, Huanghuai plain, the local government has adopted radical treatment for four consecutive years since 2007. Targeted populations with high coverage were suggested to ensure success of the strategy (Yang and Zhou, 2015). To achieve this goal requires good planning followed up by implementation which includes detailed scheduling, adequate supplies, well trained personnel, awareness and involvement of targeted communities. CDC staffs or village health workers were involved in the process of drug administration. "Distribute drugs and water to the individual's hand, watch them finish taking drugs and do not leave until drugs are swallowed"was the requirement during the implementation. For the adverse side effects, directly observed the therapy was used during the daily administration of medications to ensure safety of the treatment intervention. In the daily house visits, individuals were questioned about adverse effects of the treatment taken the previous day. A decision would then be made by health workers on whether the next dose should be given. In 2007 alone, a total of 80,438 residents were treated in spring, including those who had a history of *vivax* malaria episode in the previous year, their family members, their neighbouring household residents, and all villagers from the high incidence villages (Zhang et al., 2008; Zhou et al., 2009b). The targets shifted from a broad coverage of the population to specific at risk communities, with the change of malaria burden, radical treatment changed to targeting individuals were infected *P. vivax* or *Plasmodium ovale* (*P. ovale*) within the last year currently.

3.3.3 Vector control

Biological control: Biological control is the introduction of natural predators of *Anopheles* into larval habitats (WHO, 2019), including predatory fish, predatory invertebrates and parasites, or other disease-causing organisms. You et al. (1993) introduced tropical wicker fish to mosquito breeding sites and then evaluated the mosquito-killing effects. They found that wicker fish not only successfully survive overwinter, but also have a breeding period of more than half a year and have a good control effect on *Anopheles* larvae in various breeding sites.

Chemical control: Since the 1970s, insecticide-treated bed nets (ITNs) have been used as one of the main strategies for vector control in Henan Province, particularly pyrethroid insecticides such as deltamethrin. Bai Qiang et al. found that the density of *An. anthropophagens* and *An. Sinensis* decreased significantly after deltamethrin ITNs distributed in Shihe and Pingqiao county (Bai et al., 2003). In addition, the usage of 5% deltamethrin ITNs for two consecutive years at malaria outbreak sites resulted in a reduction of vector density, no *An. Anthropophagens* were captured, and the density of *An. sinensis* decreased sharply too, the prevalence of *Plasmodium* infections was 0, decreased by 94.90%(Zhong et al., 1998).

In 1995, local outbreaks occurred in Tongbai, Tanghe, Shihe and Pingqiao counties in the Tongbai Mountains. As *An. anthropophagus* was the main vector of the regions, from 1996 to 1998 and 2000, ITNs were distributed to the residents and then local outbreaks were controlled rapidly, the prevalence of *vivax* infections in 2003 decreased 90.06% compared to 1995 (Xu et al., 2011).

3.3.4 Capacity building

To improve malaria surveillance and ensure the professional skills of those involved in malaria prevention and control, many training courses were conducted every year. Provincial CDC conducted training on malaria epidemiological investigation, vector surveillance, control measures and strategies for personnel in district and county CDCs; provide professional training on malaria microscopy for microscopy personnel. District and county CDC conducted annual training on malaria diagnosis and treatment for doctors in health institutions in their counties and townships, as well as professional training on microscopy.

4. Case studies on implementation of One Health approach in malaria control in Henan Province

4.1 Response to malaria re-emergence in Yongcheng county

Yongcheng county, located in the easternmost part of the Huanghuai plain and surrounded by Anhui Province to the South, East and North. Historically Yongcheng had been suffered from vivax malaria epidemic transmitted by *An. sinensis* mosquitoes, with the highest malaria incidence of 33.68% in 1970. The malaria incidence was less than 1 per 10,000and reached the standard of "virtually malaria elimination" in 1991 (Zhang et al., 2006a). At the beginning of this century, Yongcheng experienced a significant re-emergence of malaria with 2890 cases reported in 2006, accounted for 56.78% of the cases in whole province, and 262.73 times than that in 1991. Furthermore, 36 outbreak foci were found in four townships. Local government paid more attention to such a severe re-emergence of malaria in Yongcheng county. A series of "extraordinary" measures were adopted to control the rapid growth of the malaria situation in Yongcheng (Zhou et al., 2018b).

Strengthen leadership and increasing investment: A lead group of malaria control had been established to provide overall leadership and direction for malaria control, which was headed by the mayor of the Yongcheng government. Commitment letter for malaria control was signed by local governments in 29 townships. Since 2007, the Yongcheng government has allocated annual 800,000 RMB of special funds to ensure malaria control.

Strengthen the treatment and management of cases: The local CDC attaches great importance to the early detection and the standard treatment of malaria patients. Anti-malarial drugs were distributed to village doctors for timely treatment. To ensure that every malaria patient receives regular treatment, village doctors are required to deliver drugs to patients and supervise them take the drugs day by day.

Strengthening training: Technicians at county/township levels were given training and retraining to improve the capacity of malaria control measures. Village doctors were given training courses of malaria for timely diagnosis and standard treatment.

MDA of radical treatment: In addition to conventional radical treatment, which give primaquine 8 times in 8 days to the *vivax* malaria patients in next spring season, MDA of radical treatment (chloroquine/primaquine 8 times in 8 days) were given to all residents of in 4 townships with outbreak foci in 2007 (Zhou et al., 2009b). 2890 cases were reported in 2006, 96.49% (80,438/83,357) of residents were given the radical treatment, and 96.40% (80,050/80,438) of which were given standard treatment.

Biological larvicides of vector control measures: Biological larvicides of *Bacillus sphaericus (Bs)* were used in 31 administrative villages with the border of Anhui Province every 15 days to reduce the density of *An. sinensis*.

Health promotion and community participation: Under the guidance of Health Administrative Department, all kinds of material such as slogans, leaflets, posters, billboards and traditional paper folding for local populations to provide health education about malaria control and prevention information. Simultaneously, publicity calendars, manuals, and cards with malaria messages were given to residents with high incidence by house-to-house, to enhance malaria knowledge such as prevention, diagnosis and treatment among high-risk population.

Improving the analysis of data and early warning system: In order to facilitate prompt notification of the status of the malaria epidemic to higher administrative departments, Yongcheng CDC paid more attention to analysis of the case reports and trends of malaria dynamics daily. Analysis and early warning of malaria reports (Ten-day report of malaria situation) were given to local government every 10 days.

Co-operation and achievements of malaria control: In the face of malaria re-emergence, Yongcheng government has integrated different departments and titanic efforts to strengthen the intervention measures related to climate, bodies of water, agriculture, mosquito vectors, and human factors. After the implementation of these package measures, the re-emergence was controlled successfully. 1579 malaria cases were reported in 2007, a decrease of 45.36% compared with previous year, and kept decreasing trend year by year, then achieved no indigenous cases reported by 2012 (Chen et al., 2019).

4.2 The conversion of dry land to lotus ponds stimulated malaria outbreak

Shangshui county, located in south-eastern Henan Province, was an endemic area of *vivax* malaria transmitted by *An. sinensis* mosquitoes, With great efforts, Shangshui reached the standard of "basic malaria elimination" in 1989 (Hao et al., 2004), and no malaria cases reported in the county from 1993 to 1997. But a local outbreak was induced by malaria patient returning from Yunnan Province in 1998 (Hao and Dou, 2005), who was not given timely treatment. From a One Health perspective, a multidisciplinary approach investigating human, environmental, and vector factors has been carried out.

Field investigation: Malaria prevalence increased following this local outbreak, from 1 patient in 1998, 8 patients in 1999, to 497 patients in 2000. From June 30 to July 2, 2001, 7808 residents were interviewed in 9 administrative villages in 3 townships, and 347 had a history of malaria, with an incidence of 4.44%. From July 4 to 6, 81 febrile patients and 265 primary school students were screened, 13 and 5 were detected as *P. vivax* positive, respectively. 75 *An. sinensis* were captured outdoors under human nets from 20:00 to 21:00 at the site.

Risk factors: Most residents in the region have bed nets, the coverage rate was 50–80%during periods of high mosquito abundance. Insecticide has also be employed, with the usage rate of 30–50%, went up to 80% in some village. Most of villages have been surrounded by rivers, and a great scale of lotus pond were converted from dry land, which were suitable breeding sites for *An. sinensis*, drastically increasing vector density.

Analysis for possible reasons of the outbreak: A combination of factors contributed to this malaria outbreak, but the change of the environment, in which dry land was converted to lotus ponds maybe the main factor. These ponds served as reservoirs for stagnant water, caused a large increase in the vector mosquitoes density (Chen et al., 2004).

Environmental modification and achievements: After strengthening early detection, standard treatment, MDA of radical treatment in the outbreak sites, and converting lotus ponds back into dry land, the local outbreak was effectively controlled. 262 malaria cases were reported and malaria incidence was reduced to 2.27/10,000 in 2002, with remarked decline of 85.26% than that in last year.

4.3 Outbreak of *Falciparum* malaria from migrant population in Taikang county

On the morning of August 23, 1997, some patients had fever and symptoms similar to malaria were reported at the Health Centre of Changying

Township, Taikang county. Taikang was in the eastern of Henan Province and reached the standard of "basic malaria elimination" in 1991. All the patients were migrant workers returning from Hainan Province, the county health department attached great importance to it and immediately conduct a special investigation.

Basic information: Changying Township has 36 administrative villages, 81 natural villages, and total population was 62,636. At the time of the outbreak, no malaria cases had occurred in the townships or its surrounding counties since 1992. 168 residents had just returned (Aug.18-Aug.22) from Dongfang City, Hainan Province, where malaria is endemic. The migrant workers had been living and staying in Dongfang City for about 6–52 days. An survey was performed to the 168 migrant workers at once, and 41 were *falciparum* malaria positive, account for 24.40%.

Analysis of infection association among cases: The date of onset of the first case was on Aug.18, 1997 and the date of onset of the latest case was on Aug.22, 1997. The interval was 4 days between the first case and the latest one. There was residence history at constructing site of all 41patients. Two generations of transmission in these cluster cases was not possible because about 1 month interval for 2 generations' transmission was required.

Analysis of possible infection sites: According to the investigation and analysis of the living locations and activity trail of the 41 cases, all these 41 cases had been living and staying in Dongfang City within 1 month before the onset, and Dongfang City might be the co-exposure site for these cases, with the following two possible sources of infection: First, malaria was endemic in Dongfang City, but Taikang county reached the standard of "basic malaria elimination" in 1991 and no *falciparum* malaria reported historically. Second, the workers lived and stay outside overnight without anti-mosquito facility, thus, this increased probability of contact with *Anopheles* mosquitoes as well as populations.

Focus disposal: All cases were treated with pyronaridine phosphate, 127 negative migrant workers, 368 family members and 492 neighbours were given extended treatment. In addition, all fever patients without defined reasons of fever were tested with blood smear examination. Meantime, malaria promotion leaflets were distributed, malaria promotion posters were posted to improve residents' health awareness.

Achievements: The implementation of these measures resulted in the rapid control of the outbreak of imported *falciparum* malaria in Taikang county. No secondary cases were reported in the surrounding population during 2 years of observation after the outbreak.

5. Introduction of malaria control technologies supported by One Health approach

5.1 Genetic tracking of *Vivax* malaria

WHO certification of malaria elimination in a country requires proof that local transmission of all human malaria parasites has been interrupted, resulting in zero indigenous cases for at least the past three consecutive years (WHO, 2017). Thus, distinguishing local from imported cases has become critical in malaria elimination. The current method of distinguishing between locally infected and imported cases is based solely on the patients' travel history, and this poses a major risk to the achievement of malaria elimination goals. Therefore, the establishment of genetic epidemiology is the most urgent in the malaria elimination phase.

The *P. vivax* circumsporozoite (CSP) gene is a well-studied molecular marker that is widely used in genotyping studies (Xu et al., 2010).CSP is mainly found on the surface of *P. vivax* sporozoites and is involved in the motility and invasion of the sporozoite during its entrance in the hepatocyte (Kappe et al., 2004; Mota and Rodriguez, 2004). The entire protein can be segmented into three regions: the N-terminal region containing a conserved pentapeptide; the central repeat region with species specificity consisting of 15–21 nonapeptide repeats (Liu et al., 2014a); and the C-terminal region containing another conserved sequence (Plassmeyer et al., 2009). The type and number of repeats in central region varies widely depending on the geographical distribution of the strain.

The study about the CSP genes of all *vivax* malaria cases in Henan Province since 2011 (Liu et al., 2018) showed that 600–750 bp bands were amplified in all cases and that the CSP sequences were significantly different between indigenous and imported cases. The number of central repeat units of the local CSP sequence ranged from 20 to 22, and an insertion sequence of 12 amino acids could be seen after the central repeat region, while the number of the imported isolates ranged from 17 to 19. Genotyping is a useful tool to determine the origin of *vivax* malaria and discriminate imported cases from indigenous cases (Liu et al., 2015). This is very significant in the elimination era.

5.2 Bacterial larvicides for malaria control in Yongcheng county

In 2003, after 11 consecutive years of no local malaria cases reported, local malaria cases reappeared in Yongcheng county due to the influence of surrounding areas. By 2006, 36 outbreaks had appeared in four townships

(Zhou et al., 2008). Yongcheng county is an area with *An. sinensis* distribution, and the local malaria prevention and control strategy focused on strengthening infectious source control and vector control measures to reduce the incidence (Zhang et al., 2007). Due to the widespread distribution of *An. sinensis* and the ineffectiveness of indoor and outdoor residual spraying, no significant progress has been made against vector control in the area. In response to malaria outbreak, besides conventional malaria control measures such as standardizing the management of malaria patients, 31 administrative villages which experienced malaria outbreaks in 2006 implemented larval source management with *Bs.* for the first time in Henan Province.

All stages of *An. sinensis* larvae were visible on the second day after *Bs.* spraying, but only the first instar larvae were visible on the 14th day. Larval density decreased by 75.6% and 76.2% after the first and third sprays, respectively, and by 100% after the fourth spraying. The density of adult *An. sinensis* also decreased by 64% and 50% after the first and third sprays, respectively, and the density of adult mosquitoes decreased to 0 after the fourth spraying. Larval and adult mosquitoes decreased by 32.4% and 14.3%, respectively, on the second day after the second spraying when rain occurred that night (Zhou et al., 2009a).

The effect of Bacterial larvicides control measures was evaluated. Compared to 2006, malaria incidence in the treated villages in 2007 decreased by 51.02%, while 40.0% in the control villages (Zhou et al., 2009a). It suggests larviciding is an effective intervention against malaria, and it can be applied to control malaria re-emergence in other areas.

6. One Health approach applied in prevention of malaria retransmission

6.1 Surveillance of imported cases

All health institutions shave facilitated with malaria laboratory diagnosis capabilities. For patients with "three kinds of fevers" (before 2015, it refers to typical malaria clinical symptoms, atypical symptoms, and fever of unknown origin) or people with suspected malaria (after 2015, refers to people with a history of living in a country where malaria is endemic, or a history of blood transfusion in the past 2 weeks, or a history of malaria in the past and patients with unexplained fever), adopt microscopic examination or rapid diagnostic test (RDT). From 2012 to 2018, the total number of malaria parasite testing (microscopic examination or RDT testing) was 4,813,663, and 1294 cases were confirmed step by step, with a positive rate of

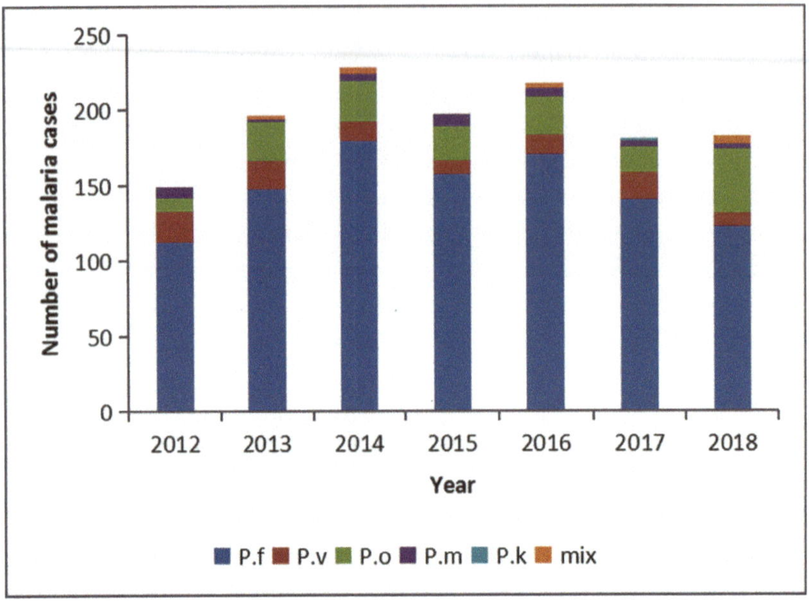

Fig. 4 *Plasmodium* species of malaria cases in Henan Province from 2012 to 2018. Abbreviation: *P. f*=*Plasmodium falciparum*, *P. v*=*Plasmodium vivax*, *P. o*=*Plasmodium ovale*, *P. m*=*Plasmodium malariae*, *P. k*=*Plasmodium knowlesi*, mix=mixed infection (Zhang et al., 2020).

0.03%, including 991 *P. falciparum* cases, 100 *P. vivax* cases, 157 *P. ovale* cases, 36 *P. malariae* cases, 9 mixed infection cases, and 1 *Pheidole knowlesi* case (Zhou et al., 2018a) (Fig. 4).

The Entry-exit inspection and quarantine also use microscopic examination or RDT on imported fever cases from malaria endemic areas, and send the blood samples of confirmed cases to CDC for confirmation, 126,642 persons were examined, and 18 malaria cases were detected from 2011 to 2014 (Wang et al., 2016).

6.2 Management of imported cases

In 2004, China completed the Chinese Information System for Disease Control and Prevention (CISDCP). CDCs at the county level and above, medical institutions at the county level and above, and community-level medical and health institutions have the capacity to report the cases of the notifiable infectious diseases in real time by this web-based system. Malaria, as a national category B notifiable infectious disease, is required to be reported directly online within 24h after case detection. In 2011, the "Malaria Subsystem" was added to the web-based system entitled

"National Information Management System for Parasitic Disease Control". In addition to the basic information on malaria cases reported directly on the internet, the information on epidemiological investigation of malaria cases, investigation and disposal of epidemic focus, malaria surveillance and other related information were added.

In order to avoid local reintroduction of malaria, the"1–3-7"approach was implemented in Henan Province, with a core of tracking and identifying the source of infection. The"1"in the"1–3–7" approach means that within 1 day (24 h), all malaria cases must be reported to the CISDCP. "3" refers to the completion of case confirmation and epidemiology investigation within 3 days. And"7"means that within 7 days, the loci of the reported cases should be investigated and respond with vector control and health advocacy measures. The completion status of Henan's malaria elimination "1-3-7" strategy during 2012–2018 is shown in Table 1 (Zhang et al., 2020).

6.3 Treatment of imported cases

General and specialized hospitals at all levels are responsible for malaria cases treatment. All laboratory-confirmed malaria cases should be treated with appropriate anti-malarial drugs as described in "Guideline for Anti-malarial Drugs in China (WS/T 485-2016)".

To strengthen the treatment of severe malaria and reduce deaths, Henan Provincial Health Department designated "Henan Provincial Infectious Disease Hospital" as the provincial designated hospital for malaria treatment

Table 1 The "1-3-7" approach to malaria surveillance and response in Henan Province during 2012–2018 (Zhang et al., 2020).

Year	Total No. of cases	No. of cases reported within 1 day (%)	No. of cases investigated within 3 days (%)	No. of foci investigated within 7 days (%)
2012	156	156 (100)	155 (99.4)	156 (100)
2013	197	197 (100)	196 (99.5)	197 (100)
2014	216	216 (100)	213 (98.6)	216 (100)
2015	184	184 (100)	183 (99.5)	184 (100)
2016	198	198 (100)	196 (99.0)	198 (100)
2017	169	169 (100)	169 (100)	96 (56.8)
2018	174	174 (100)	172 (98.9)	165 (94.8)
Total	1294	1294 (100)	1284 (99.2)	1212 (93.7)

Table 2 Results of three methods in malaria reference laboratory of Henan Province from 2015 to 2019 (Li et al., n.d.).

	Microscopy (detective rate/%)	PCR (detective rate/%)	RDT (detective rate/%)	Final diagnosis
P. falciporum	721	807	830	820
P. vivax	58	64		64
P. malariae	32	35		35
P. ovale	146	141		148
P. knowlesi	1	1		1
Mixed	1	10		10
Positive	1	6	215	
Negative	202	125	144	116
Others	32	5	5	
Total	1194	1194	1194	1194

in 2010, it was also the first designated hospital for malaria treatment in China. In 2018, 27 more hospitals designated for malaria treatment in 17 municipalities and 10 counties, so that the severe cases can be rescued nearby.

From 2012 to 2018, a total of 865 in-patient malaria cases were treated across the province, including 208 severe malaria cases, all of which were imported *falciparum* malaria, and 12 cases died during hospitalization.

6.4 Reference laboratory network

Reference laboratory network for malaria is composed of provincial reference laboratory, municipal and county–level CDC and medical facilities at all levels of Henan Province. Medical facilities are eligible for malaria diagnosis, to perform laboratory testing and identification of malaria parasites. County and municipal CDC are responsible for the case review, training and quality control, etc. County CDC are responsible for microscopic examination and review of all positive blood smears and no less than 10% negative blood smears collected from the medical facilities in the county; municipal CDC are responsible for rechecking all positive blood smears and no less than 3% negative blood smears for each county every year. Provincial reference laboratory is responsible for case confirmation, training, quality control, technical support and evaluation, establishing malaria case information database to enable the exchange and sharing of relevant information, carrying out research on new technologies and new methods related to malaria diagnosis (Fig. 5). By now, 3 microscopists obtained level 1 certificates, 2 obtained level 2 certificates in Henan Province, which were awarded by WHO.

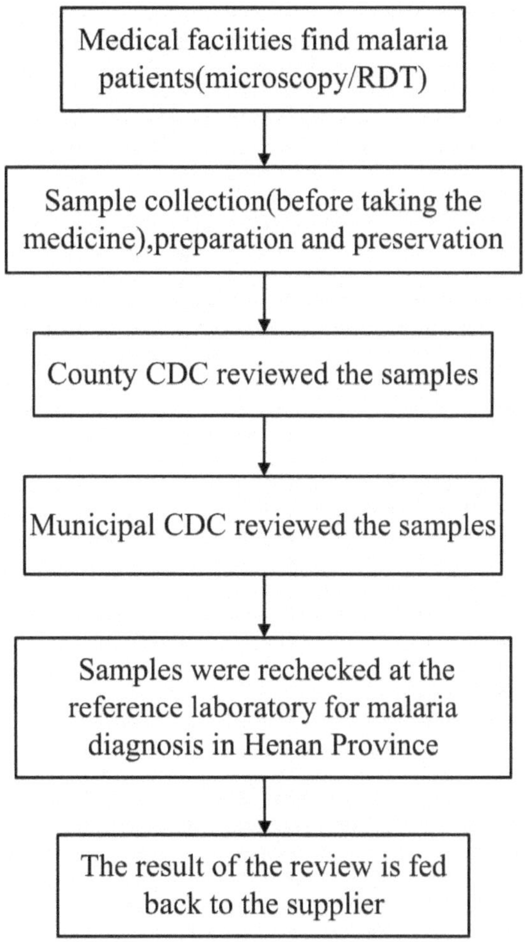

Fig. 5 Malaria diagnosis review network in Henan Province. From 2015 to 2019, Henan provincial reference laboratory for malaria received a total of 1194 samples, and then reviewed by microscopy, RDT and PCR methods simultaneously, 1078malaria cases were confirmed finally. The laboratory-confirmed cases consisted of 820 *P. falciparum* (76.07%), 64 *P. vivax* (5.94%), 35 *P. malariae* (3.25%), 148 *P. ovale* (13.73%), 1 *Pheidole knowlesi* (0.09%), 10 mixed infection cases (0.93%) (Table 2) (Li et al., n.d.).

6.5 Entomological surveillance and vector control

6.5.1 Entomological surveillance

During the malaria elimination stage, vector surveillance is performed to provide a scientific basis for correctly determining the type of epidemic focus and implementing corresponding vector control measures. According to different locations, 17 malaria vector sentinel sites were established in the Henan Province, which together form the provincial malaria vector surveillance network with annual vector population monitoring. In addition to annual surveillance, additional vector investigations are performed under certain circumstances, such as epidemic areas with imported *vivax* malaria cases but without vector investigations during the past 3 years. On-site investigation of imported re-transmission is also performed. According to the vector population monitoring results, *An. sinensis* has been found at all the sentinel sites. *An. yatsushiroensis* and *An. lesteri* have also been detected at some sites (Zhang et al., 2015). In 2010 and 2011, Liu et al. applied the "mark-release-recapture" technique for the first time in China to study the flight distance of *An. sinensis*, and found that the recapture rate of *An. sinensis* was low, the maximum flight distance was 400 m, and most of them were recaptured within a radius of 100 m from the release point (Liu et al., 2011).

6.5.2 Monitoring insecticide resistance

The wide use of insecticides has allowed for effective control of malaria and has thereby benefited human health. However, as a consequence to this intervention, developed insecticide resistance among vector species has become a concern (Su et al., 2019). Insecticide resistance is the ability of mosquitoes to survive exposure to a standard dose of insecticide, owing to physiological or behavioural adaptations (WHO, 2016). The emergence and increase of resistance not only reduced the utility of currently available insecticides but also undermines the efficacy of newly discovered or developed insecticides, causing ecological, environmental, and human health problems (Cui et al., 2006). Therefore, insecticide resistance monitoring in vector mosquitoes is essential to guide the rational use of insecticides in vector control programmes (Qin et al., 2014; Xu et al., 2014). According to "Test methods of mosquito resistance to insecticides—Bioassay methods" (GB/T 26347-2010) (MOH, 2011), insecticidal susceptibility is determined by the WHO recommended insecticide-susceptibility test. The susceptibility of *An. sinensis* to malathion, deltamethrin and lambda-cyhalothrin were investigated in Puyang County in 2018 and 2020 (Hu et al., 2021), and the results showed that the half knockdown times (KT_{50}) of malathion were 91.08 and 40.95 min, with 60-min knockdown rates of 37.50% and 60.87% and 24-h mortality rates of 90.91% and 100%, indicating that the resistance levels of malathion were moderately resistant (M) and susceptible (S), respectively. The insecticide resistance levels of deltamethrin and lambda-cyhalothrin were found to be resistant (R) in the 2 years through the same index. The results indicated that *An. sinensis* is relatively susceptible to malathion but has developed high-level resistance to deltamethrin and lambda-cyhalothrin in Puyang county, Henan Province.

6.5.3 Vector control

Vector control measures were implemented in combination with Patriotic Health Campaign and New Rural Construction, which successfully mobilized people to improve environmental sanitation and change health behaviours. Under the extensive long-term implementation of comprehensive vector control measures, the breeding environment of *anopheles* changed, thus reducing their distribution range, decreasing or eliminating their populations, weakening the intensity of malaria transmission and changing the conditions of malaria transmission in some areas.

In this stage of malaria elimination, indoor residual spraying (IRS) has been mainly used in the focus where transmission has occurred or with potential for transmission. In the potential transmission focus, IRS is used in key areas to eliminate suspected infected adult mosquitoes. The insecticides used in IRS are mainly pyrethroids, such as beta-cyfluthrin suspension concentrate and beta-cypermethrin suspension concentrate. From 2011 to 2018, 35,500 kg of insecticides was purchased for ITNs, and the population protected by IRS across the Henan Province has reached 160,346.

6.6 Public health education and health promotion

6.6.1 National Malaria Day

Under the guidance of Health Administrative Department, and combining with annual publicity activities of National Malaria Day on April 26, all counties across the province use slogans, leaflets, posters, audio-visual materials and traditional paper folding for local populations to provide health education about malaria control and prevention information. Simultaneously, for the multi-sectoral department cooperation, malaria control and prevention information can be spread through newspapers, radio, television and other communication media. In recent years, new online media such as Wechat and Weibo become very popular in China and have been used to spread and propagandize a variety of malaria information.

6.6.2 Innovative forms of health education

Besides the conventional ways of health promotion, all levels of CDCs had innovated methods to provide malaria prevention and control information. Clear guidelines in the language understood by local residents, posters, wall charts, educational videos and other teaching materials can improve the understanding of malaria. Such as the local operas "Return from Africa" and "Business Travel," created, directed, and performed by CDC staffs by themselves, welcomed by the general public. These will increase the likelihood of better prescribing and adherence. In addition, health education was also did in school, named "Children Lead Parents," as whatever the children learned in school about malaria knowledge, good sanitation and healthy lifestyles will be carried back to their families and their communities. In many parts of the world, schoolchildren have proved to be very good teachers to their family members who have not had the benefit of instruction in the basic lessons in healthy living.

6.6.3 "Two letters and one commitment"

To improve both health workers' and high-risk populations' awareness, "Two Letters and One Commitment" activities were taken across the entire province. These activities consisted of a letter to migrant workers abroad, a letter to clinicians, and a letter of commitment from village doctors. To tell them that if there are patients returning from malaria endemic areas of Africa and Southeast Asia with unexplained fever, then they should consider checking for malaria *Plasmodium*. These activities significantly enhance awareness of malaria among high-risk populations and health care providers.

6.6.4 Health promotion in specific populations

Most Chinese citizens who travel to malaria-endemic countries are workers and technicians, they usually stay in malaria-endemic areas for a long time. At present, there is currently no suitable prophylactic drugs for them. Therefore, Henan Province has mainly adopted health education practices to prevent malaria in this population by recommending the use of anti-mosquito facilities and products for disease prevention. CDCs at all levels cooperate with relevant departments as well as relevant overseas engineering companies to train accompanying doctors on malaria diagnosis and treatment skills, and to conduct malaria prevention and control education to prevent mosquito bites and improve vector control skills for overseas personnel. Taking advantage of the yellow fever vaccine requirements for people travelling to Africa, customs agents carry out malaria protection knowledge education in its subordinate international travel health centres at all levels through electronic LED display screen or distribution malaria materials such as posters or leaflets, provide free consultation and laboratory testing for fever after returning home.

6.7 Research on socio-economic factors

Malaria is not only an infectious disease transmitted by mosquitoes but also a social disease influenced by human activities and economic status. Human awareness and behaviour have a certain impact on malaria transmission. Zhuang et al. (1997) evaluated the quality and effectiveness of malaria control measures in low-endemic areas from the economic perspective in Henan Province, indicating that if government investment decrease, malaria burden would increase, causing delays in treatment, and then leading to accumulation of infectious sources. To understand the costs and factors associated with the diagnosis and treatment of malaria, surveys were investigated and analysed in Henan Province from November 2013 to October 2014 (Liu et al., 2016). The median amount of money spent on malaria in urban subgroup was 4833 RMB, which is approximately triple of that in rural subgroup, while the median amount of money spent on malaria in the province was 2000 RMB. The highest cost was 92,000 RMB, which far exceeds the mean annual income of rural residents in Henan Province of 8475.3 RMB (NBS, 2014). The cost is related to the level of medical institutions visited (Sun et al., 2009; Tang et al., 2017). In comparison, the patients confirmed in CDC spent lease money.

In view of this, training to improve skill and awareness of medical institutions is required.

7. Lessons learnt from malaria control and elimination in Henan Province

7.1 Attentions of governments at all levels were paid, which provided organizational foundation and facilitated the actions on malaria elimination

Under the unified leadership of provincial government as well as governments at all levels, the multi-department cooperation mechanism was built and implemented. In 2010, 13 departments including the former Bureau of

Health jointly issued the Henan Malaria Elimination Action Plan (2010–2020), clearly requires all the departments to cooperate closely and jointly perform their duties to achieve malaria elimination. The Development and Reform Commission and Department of Finance are responsible for including malaria elimination programme in the Provincial Economic and Social Development Plan, arranging for special funds for malaria control and elimination, and strengthening fund supervision. The departments of customs, public security, tourism, commerce cooperate with the Health departments to provide malaria health education, case surveillance and disease prevention management for entry-exit population, and share the information with the health departments in a timely manner. Radio and television administrations are responsible for arranging various forms of malaria prevention and control education. The Bureau of Education is responsible for health education on malaria prevention and control in primary and secondary schools. Bureau of Scientific and Technological has included scientific research projects on malaria control and elimination as part of the provincial science and technology plan.

7.2 Efficient mechanism of multi-regional joint control promoted malaria elimination in grand regions at large

Cross-regional malaria joint prevention and control was proved to be a successful mechanism to promote the cross-regional control goals involving multiple neighbouring areas with similar geography characteristics, socio-economic characteristics, malaria epidemic modes, and epidemic intensity. Henan Province has participated regional cooperation since 1974. The multi-regional joint control has established a province annual rotation duty, cross-check and annual meeting mechanism. The provinces on duty in turn are responsible for regional cooperation of malaria elimination and prevention re-establishment including cross-checks and annual meeting, etc. At the same time, the advanced experience and lessons can be shared with each other through cross-checks and annual meeting.

7.3 Comprehensive control measures acted as an important role in malaria control

Over past decades, a wide variety of comprehensive and strict prevention and control measures were implemented towards malaria control and elimination, according to various epidemic and local conditions. According to the biological and transmission dynamics of different vectors, specific malaria control strategies were implemented in areas with different vector distribution.

For example, an integrated prevention and control strategy, primarily involving infectious source management, was used in *P. vivax* endemic areas with *An. sinensis* as the main vector. *An. Sinensis* has the characteristic of mammalophilic, both campestral and domesticity and IRS is incompletely effectiveness. A strategy that paid equal attention to the vector control and infection source management was used in malaria-endemic areas with *An. anthropophagus* as the main vector. *An. Anthropophagus* has the characteristic of anthropophilic, domesticity, transmitting both *P. falciparum* and *P. vivax*, and IRS is effective. In the elimination stage, the priority of malaria elimination transformed from population-based intervention to case (focus) intervention as core, thus facilitating the implementation of malaria elimination across the province.

7.4 Scientific researches on this field provided strong support to malaria elimination

A great deal of attentions has been paid to scientific research on malaria prevention and control in Henan Province from the very beginning of malaria control programme. Such as a series of laboratory studies and field operational researches on malaria elimination strategies and key technologies including the pathogenic biology of malaria, vector biology, diagnostics, antimalarial drugs, control strategies, etc. The study about the long and short incubation of *P. vivax* confirmed that the ratio of the long and short incubation in Henan is about 3:1. To evaluate the effect of chloroquine-primaquine, studies of 3-day, 5-day, and 8-day intermittent therapy were carried out successively, and it was determined that 8-day therapy is the most appropriate, providing a scientific evidence for these lection of treatment strategy. A biological study of the vector showed that *An. anthropophagus* is the main vector within its distribution areas. Genetic tracking of *vivax* malaria was used to determine the source of imported *P. vivax* malaria infection successfully. The timely transformation and application of scientific research results have lifted the level of science and technology on malaria elimination.

7.5 Risks for re-establishment of malaria

Examples of resurgence caused by imported cases happened frequently in areas without local transmission worldwide, for instance, the resurgence in Shangshui County. After malaria elimination has been achieved, a programme for the prevention of re-establishment should continue until malaria eradicational over the world. Such a programme should be integrated into public health programmes to maintain the necessary technical expertise, even if the responsible staff no longer work solely on malaria. On the basis of the original "1–3–7" approaches, strong surveillance and early warnings of disease outbreak, combined with multi-departmental cooperation mechanisms, timely and proper diagnosis and treatment of the imported cases, and investigation and evaluation of the risk of malaria re-introduction should be conducted to prevent re-establishment of malaria transmission.

8. Conclusions and perspectives

8.1 Conclusions

Malaria was an infectious disease with the longest history, the largest influence, and the most serious destructions in Henan Province. Malaria not only seriously endangered the health and property of people but also affected economic and social development in the region. After arduous efforts over more than seven decades, malaria prevention, control, and diagnostic capabilities have been significantly improved, disease burden has been dramatically reduced. Henan Province achieved the goal of eliminating malaria throughout the province in 2019. This achievement was due to the establishment of an effective cross-sectoral, coordinated government unit, a regional joint-control mechanism, a sensitive surveillance system for case detection, an enhanced workforce trained for all kinds of abilities, extensive health education activities involving community participation, and a productive public health scientific programme. The entire process of malaria control and elimination in Henan Province is based on the multi-sectoral, cross-regional, and multidisciplinary One Health approach (Munyua et al., 2019). The adoption of the One Health approach in Henan Province has led to rapid response and control of malaria outbreaks and has thereby promoted provincial malaria elimination.

8.2 Perspectives

Although China has achieved the goal of malaria elimination, it still remains to be a common challenge facing the world at large. There is a long way to go to malaria eradication worldwide, and no country can afford to remain apathetic in this matter. In the face of unprecedented global changes, China should actively promote and lead the construction of a "One health" approach. Experts in public health, zoology, and environmental science should work together with many functional departments to build a multi-party cooperation and coordination mechanism to adapt to the current situation of malaria prevention and control. The former "passive response mode" aimed at safeguarding local economic interests should be transformed into an "active response mode" aimed at protecting human health. International cooperation and exchanges should be strengthened, and normalized cooperation between countries will be established based on platforms such as the Belt and Road Initiative, to contribute to a community of shared future for human health.

Acknowledgements

This work was supported by the Bill & Melinda Gates Foundation (No. INV-018913).

References

Aguirre, A.A., Longcore, T., Barbieri, M., Dabritz, H., Hill, D., Klein, P.N., Lepczyk, C., Lilly, E.L., McLeod, R., Milcarsky, J., et al., 2019. The one health approach to toxoplasmosis: epidemiology, control, and prevention strategies. EcoHealth 16, 378–390.

Bai, Q., Yang, Z.Y., Yuan, F.R., Dai, X.J., Liu, J.L., 2003. Effection of malaria control with deltamethrin suspension-treated nets. Chin. J. Parasit. Dis. Con. 16, 73.

Baum, E., Sattabongkot, J., Sirichaisinthop, J., Kiattibutr, K., Davies, D.H., Jain, A., Lo, E., Lee, M.C., Randall, A.Z., Molina, D.M., et al., 2015. Submicroscopic and asymptomatic plasmodium falciparum and plasmodium vivax infections are common in western Thailand—molecular and serological evidence. Malar. J. 14, 95.

Chen, J.S., Li, P., Shang, L.Y., Li, X.H., Zhao, J.H., 2004. Investigation on epidemic factors of malaria outbreak in Shangshui County. Henan J. Prev. Med. 15, 153–155.

Chen, C.W., Guan, Z., Gao, C.Q., Zhu, L., Shen, Y., Zhang, H.W., Liu, Y., 2019. Malaria epidemiological characteristics in Yongcheng, Henan, 2007-2017. China Trop. Med. 19, 386–388.

Cornille-Brögger, R., Mathews, H.M., Storey, J., Ashkar, T.S., Brögger, S., Molineaux, L., 1978. Changing patterns in the humoral immune response to malaria before, during, and after the application of control measures: a longitudinal study in the west African savanna. Bull. World Health Organ. 56, 579–600.

Cui, F., Raymond, M., Qiao, C.L., 2006. Insecticide resistance in vector mosquitoes in China. Pest Manag. Sci. 62, 1013–1022.

Guo, W.S., Zhao, D.Y., Zhang, H.W., Lu, D.L., Liu, Y., Qian, D., Yang, C.Y., Guan, Z., Zhao, Y.L., Zhou, R.M., et al., 2021. Epidemiological characteristics of malaria in Henan Province from 1950 to 2019. Chin. J. Schisto Control 33, 62–65.

Hao, J.L., Dou, C.Y., 2005. Investigation report on malaria incidence and epidemic trend in Shangshui county, 1998–2003. Pract. Prevent. Med. 12, 353.

Hao, J.L., Wu, W.M., Dou, C.Y., 2004. Investigation and control of malaria outbreak in Shangshui county from 2001 to 2003. Chin. J. Parasitol. Parasit. Dis. 22, 333.

Hu, Y.B., He, Z.Q., Liu, Y., Qian, D., Yang, C.Y., Lu, D.L., Zhang, Q.Q., Zhang, H.W., 2021. Susceptibility of Anopheles sinensis to insecticides in Puyang City, Henan Province. Chin. J. Schisto Control 33, 501–504.

Kappe, S.H., Buscaglia, C.A., Nussenzweig, V., 2004. Plasmodium sporozoite molecular cell biology. Annu. Rev. Cell Dev. Biol. 20, 29–59.

Kong, X.L., Liu, Y., Wang, W.M., Xu, X., Li, K.J., Zhang, H.W., Li, W.D., Wang, R.B., 2016. A retrospective analysis on the effectiveness of falciparum malaria joint control in Jiangsu, Anhui and Henan provinces. China Trop. Med. 16, 986–988.

Li, P.Y., Yuan, L.H., Lu, J.H., 2018. Imperative one health strategy for the emerging infectious diseases. Infect. Dis. Info 31, 11–14.

Li, S. H., Ji, P. H., Zhou, R. M., He, Z. Q., Qian, D., Yang, C. Y., Liu, Y., Lu, D. L., Wang, H., Zhang, H. W., et al. Analysis of diagnosis capacities of malaria reference laboratories in Henan Province during 2015–2019. Chin. J. Parasitol. Parasit. Dis., 1–5, n.d.

Liu, X.Z., Xu, B.L., 2006. Malaria situation and evaluation on the control effect in Henan Province during 1990-2005. Chin. J. Parasitol. Parasit. Dis. 24, 226–229.

Liu, Y., Su, Y.P., Zhang, H.W., Jin, X.L., Chen, X.X., Shen, M.Z., Huang, G.Q., 2008. Analysis of malaria situation in five provinces of Jiangsu, Shandong, Henan, Anhui and Hubei in 2006. China Trop. Med. 8, 190–208.

Liu, X.B., Liu, Q.Y., Guo, Y.H., Jiang, J.Y., Ren, D.S., Zhou, G.C., Zheng, C.J., Zhang, Y., Liu, J.L., Li, Z.F., et al., 2011. The abundance and host-seeking behavior of culicine species (Diptera: Culicidae) and Anopheles sinensis in Yongcheng city, People's Republic of China. Parasit. Vectors 4, 221.

Liu, Y., Zhang, H.W., Zhou, R.M., Yang, C.Y., Qian, D., Zhao, Y.L., Xu, B.L., 2014a. First imported relapse case of plasmodium vivax malaria and analysis of its origin by CSP sequencing in Henan Province, China. Malar. J. 13, 448.

Liu, Y., Zhou, R.M., Lu, D.L., Liu, H., Qian, D., Zhang, H.W., 2014b. Analysis on malaria surveillance in Henan Province from 2005 to 2010. Modern Prevent. Med. 41, 1290–1292.

Liu, Y., Qian, D., Chen, W.Q., Zhou, R.M., Yang, C.Y., Zhao, Y.L., Xu, B.L., Zhang, H.W., 2015. Tracing investigation of one vivax malaria case by detecting the gene encoding circumsporozoite protein in Henan. Chin. J. Parasitol. Parasit. Dis. 33, 156–158.

Liu, Y., Zhang, Y.L., Gao, L.J., Qian, D., Yang, C.Y., Zhou, R.M., Xu, B.L., Zhang, H.W., 2016. Medical costs on malaria in Henan Province and analysis of the influential factors. Chin. J. Parasitol. Parasit. Dis. 34, 11–15.

Liu, Y., Zhou, R.M., Zhang, Y.L., Wang, D.Q., Li, S.H., Yang, C.Y., Qian, D., Zhao, Y.L., Zhang, H.W., Xu, B.L., 2018. Analysis of polymorphisms in the circumsporozoite protein gene of Plasmodium vivax isolates from Henan Province, China. Malar. J. 17, 103.

MOH, 2011. Test Methods of Mosquito Resistance to Insecticides—Bioassay Methods. Chinese Standard Press, Beijing.

Mota, M.M., Rodriguez, A., 2004. Migration through host cells: the first steps of plasmodium sporozoites in the mammalian host. Cell. Microbiol. 6, 1113–1118.

Munyua, P.M., Njenga, M.K., Osoro, E.M., Onyango, C.O., Bitek, A.O., Mwatondo, A., Muturi, M.K., Musee, N., Bigogo, G., Otiang, E., et al., 2019. Successes and challenges of the one health approach in Kenya over the last decade. BMC Public Health 19, 465.

NBS, 2014. China Statistical Yearbook 2013. China Statistics Press, Beijing, p. 176.

Nie, E.Q., Xia, Y., Wang, T., Lu, J.H., 2016. One health—a new approach to control emerging infectious diseases. J. Microb. Infect., 3–7.

Plassmeyer, M.L., Reiter, K., Shimp Jr., R.L., Kotova, S., Smith, P.D., Hurt, D.E., House, B., Zou, X., Zhang, Y., Hickman, M., et al., 2009. Structure of the plasmodium falciparum circumsporozoite protein, a leading malaria vaccine candidate. J. Biol. Chem. 284, 26951–26963.

Qin, Q., Li, Y., Zhong, D., Zhou, N., Chang, X., Li, C., Cui, L., Yan, G., Chen, X.G., 2014. Insecticide resistance of Anopheles sinensis and An. vagus in Hainan Island, a malaria-endemic area of China. Parasit. Vectors 7, 92.

Shang, L.Y., Gao, Q., Liu, X., Shen, M.Z., Huang, G.Q., 2006. Evaluation on the effect of cooperative malaria control in 5 provinces of Central China in 30 years. J. Pathogen Biol. 1, 51–53.

Shang, L.Y., Xu, B.L., Su, Y.P., 2011. Henan Malaria Epidemic and Control. 3 Zhongyuan Publishing Media Group, Zhengzhou (in Chinese).

Sougoufara, S., Doucoure, S., Backe Sembene, P.M., Harry, M., Sokhna, C., 2017. Challenges for malaria vector control in sub-Saharan Africa: resistance and behavioral adaptations in Anopheles populations. J. Vector Borne Dis. 54, 4–15.

Su, X., Guo, Y., Deng, J., Xu, J., Zhou, G., Zhou, T., Li, Y., Zhong, D., Kong, L., Wang, X., et al., 2019. Fast emerging insecticide resistance in Aedes albopictus in Guangzhou, China: alarm to the dengue epidemic. PLoS Negl. Trop. Dis. 13, e0007665.

Sun, L., Xu, L.Z., Liu, Z.M., Cheng, J., Chu, L., Wang, X.Z., Zhang, H., Zhou, C.C., Liao, T.H., Ding, Y., 2009. Investigate on the status of treatment expenses and analysis its influence factors in Shandong Province. Chin. Health Econ. 28, 17–18.

Tang, L.H., Gao, Q., 2013a. China's Malaria Control and Elimination. vol. 36 Shanghai Scientifical & Technical Publishers, Shanghai (in Chinese).

Tang, L.H., Gao, Q., 2013b. Malaria Control and Elimination in China. Shanghai Science and Technical Publishers, Shanghai.

Tang, S., Feng, D., Wang, R., Ghose, B., Hu, T., Ji, L., Wu, T., Fu, H., Huang, Y., Feng, Z., 2017. Economic burden of malaria inpatients during National Malaria Elimination Programme: estimation of hospitalization cost and its inter-province variation. Malar. J. 16, 291.

Thriemer, K., Ley, B., Bobogare, A., Dysoley, L., Alam, M.S., Pasaribu, A.P., Sattabongkot, J., Jambert, E., Domingo, G.J., Commons, R., et al., 2017. Challenges for achieving safe and effective radical cure of plasmodium vivax: a round table discussion of the APMEN vivax working group. Malar. J. 16, 141.

Voller, A., Bruce-Chwatt, L.J., 1968. Serological malaria surveys in Nigeria. Bull. World Health Organ. 39, 883–897.

Wang, Y.L., Li, X.M., Wang, J.J., 2016. To analysis entry-exit group infectious diseases during ten years in Henan ports. Henan J. Prev. Med. 27. 728–731 + 742.

WHO, 2016. Test Procedures for Insecticide Resistance Monitoring in Malaria Vector Mosquitoes. Switzerland, Geneva.

WHO, 2017. A Framework for Malaria Elimination. Switzerland, Geneva.

WHO, 2019. Guidelines for Malaria Vector Control. Switzerland, Geneva.

WHO, 2021. World Malaria Report 2021. Switzerland, Geneva.

Xu, G.Q., Zhang, Z.X., Li, N., Dai, H.J., 2010. Genotyping of plasmodium vivax in China-Myanmar border by circumsporozoite protein. Chin. J. Parasitol. Parasit. Dis. 28, 265–267.

Xu, B.L., Su, Y.P., Liu, Y., Zhang, H.W., He, L.J., Chen, J.S., 2011. Malaria evaluation on the control effect in Henan Province during 1970-2010. Henan J. Prev. Med., 321–326.

Xu, T., Zhong, D., Tang, L., Chang, X., Fu, F., Yan, G., Zheng, B., 2014. Anopheles sinensis mosquito insecticide resistance: comparison of three mosquito sample collection and preparation methods and mosquito age in resistance measurements. Parasit. Vectors 7, 54.

Yang, H.L., Zhou, H.N., 2015. Yunnan Malaria. Yunnan Science and Technology Press, Kunming.

Yang, C.Y., Qian, D., Lu, D.L., Liu, Y., Zhou, R.M., Li, S.H., Guan, Z., Zhao, Y.L., Zhang, H.W., Zhao, D.Y., et al., 2021. Malaria situation in Henan, 2011–2019. Modern Prevent. Med. 48, 393–397.

You, X.C., Song, J.D., Chen, J.S., 1993. Huanghuai plains reference wicker fish experimental research for the prevention and control of the anopheles. Chin. J. Parasit. Dis. Con. 6, 52–54.

Zhang, Y.S., 1995. Three provinces of Jiangsu, Anhui, Henan falciparum defense situation report. Chin. J. Parasitol. Parasit. Dis., 35–39.

Zhang, H.W., Su, Y.P., Liu, Y., Wang, Z.Q., Cui, J., 2006a. Analysis of malaria epidemic situation in Yongcheng of Henan Province in 2005. Int. J. Med. Parasit. Dis. 33, 119–121.

Zhang, H.W., Su, Y.P., Xu, B., l., 2006b. A review of malaria control and research in Henan Province of China. J. Pathogen Biol. 1, 64–66.

Zhang, H.W., Su, Y.P., Zhou, G.C., Liu, Y., Cui, J., Wang, Z.Q., 2007. Re-emerging malaria in Yongcheng city of Henan province. Chin. J. Vector Biol. Control 18, 42–44.

Zhang, H.W., Su, Y.P., Zhou, G.C., Zhou, S.M., Huang, F., 2008. Study on the selection of population for malaria transmission resting stage treatment in plain areas where malaria infection rising rapidly. China Trop. Med. 8. 359–360 + 392.

Zhang, H.W., Liu, Y., Hu, T., Zhou, R.M., Chen, J.S., Qian, D., Yang, C.Y., Zhao, Y.L., Li, S.H., Cui, J., et al., 2015. Knockdown resistance of Anopheles sinensis in Henan province, China. Malar. J. 14, 137.

Zhang, H.W., Zhang, Q.Q., Yang, C.Y., Qian, D., Lu, D.L., Zhao, Y.L., Zhou, R.M., Li, S.H., Wang, H., Liu, Y., 2019. Progress of malaria elimination and achievements of scientific researches in Henan province. Henan J. Prev. Med. 30, 721–725.

Zhang, Q.Q., Li, S.H., Liu, Y., Hu, Y.B., Guan, Z., Zhao, Y.L., Lu, D.L., Yang, C.Y., Zhang, H.W., Qian, D., et al., 2020. The "1-3-7" approach to malaria surveillance and response—Henan Province, China, 2012-2018. China CDC Weekly 2, 289–292.

Zhong, Y.G., Zhuang, J.T., Li, A.M., Shang, L.Y., He, L.J., Wang, W.S., Chen, G.Y., Li, D.Z., Zhong, S., Dang, Z.H., 1998. Observation on mosquito control effect with novel deltamethrin-treated nets. Chin. J. Vector Biol. Control 9, 4.

Zhou, X.-N., 2021. China declared malaria-free: a milestone in the world malaria eradication and Chinese public health. Infect. Dis. Poverty 10.

Zhou, G.C., Zhang, H.W., Sun, Y.P., Zhou, Y.S., Huang, F., 2008. Epidemiologic analysis of malaria outbreak in Yongcheng County of Henan Province in 2006. J. Trop. Med. 381–383 + 372.

Zhou, G.C., Zhang, H.W., Su, Y.P., Zhou, S.M., Huang, F., 2009a. Investigation into the results of control of malaria outbreak in Yongcheng County by biological control of mosquito larvae. China Trop. Med. 9. 228–229 + 259.

Zhou, G.C., Zhang, H.W., Su, Y.P., Zhou, S.S., Huang, F., 2009b. Evaluation of therapeutic measures of radical treatment for malaria in pre-transmission season in Yongcheng, Henan, China in 2007. J. Pathogen Biol. 4, 112–114.

Zhou, R.M., Li, S.H., Gao, L.J., Qian, D., Yang, C.Y., Liu, Y., Zhao, Y.L., Zhang, H.W., 2018a. Diagnosis and analysis of the first imported case of Plasmodium knowlesi infection in Henan Province. J. Zhengzhou Univ. (Med. Sci.) 53, 610–613.

Zhou, X.N., Xia, Z.G., Zhou, S.S., Xiao, N., 2018b. Roadmap Analysis on Malaria Elimination in China. Shanghai Scientifical & Technical Publishers, Shanghai, pp. 146–148.

Zhu, D.S., Yang, W.Z., Li, H.Z., Zheng, C.J., Gou, J.B., 2007. Analysis of characteristics of malaria incidence and measures for treatment of malaria in the periods of inactivity in the unstable areas of Central China. China Trop. Med. 7, 1281–1284.

Zhuang, J.A., Li, P., Lu, D.L., Dong, L.Y., Song, J.D., Liu, X.L., 1997. Henan rural doctors in the social and economic behavior and its impact on malaria prevention and treatment. Chin. Rural Health Serv. Administration, 55–57.

Zinsstag, J., Schelling, E., Waltner-Toews, D., Tanner, M., 2011. From "one medicine" to "one health" and systemic approaches to health and well-being. Prev. Vet. Med. 101, 148–156.

CHAPTER SIX

Research and development of traditional medicines in low- and middle-income countries: A case study of artemisinin discovery in China

Guang-qi Liu[a,b], Yan Xie[a,b], Yi-nuo Sun[a,b], Kai-xuan Zhang[a,b], Ji-yan Maa[a,b], and Yang-mu Huang[a,b,*]
[a]Department of Global Health, Peking University School of Public Health, Beijing, PR China
[b]Institute for Global Health, Peking University, Beijing, PR China
*Corresponding author: e-mail address: ymhuang@bjmu.edu.cn

Contents

1. Introduction 188
2. Global and Chinese background 189
   2.1 Global malaria burden in 1960s 189
   2.2 Urgent need during wartime 189
   2.3 China's low-resource status 190
3. Research and development history of artemisinin 191
   3.1 Establishing a cross-department and cross-region collaboration system 192
   3.2 Exploring traditional medicine by modern methods 194
   3.3 Promoting synergy through efficient information-sharing mechanisms 198
   3.4 National cooperation in overcoming challenge of artemisinin production 200
   3.5 Disclosure of artemisinin by Chinese government and scientists 204
4. Conclusions and perspectives 205
   4.1 Conclusions 205
   4.2 Perspectives 206
Acknowledgements 207
References 207

Abstract

Though traditional medicines have been developed through practice for thousands of years, limited research has discussed the research and development (R&D) pattern of traditional medicines. China's discovery of artemisinin accumulated valuable experiences to explore traditional medicine under low-resource settings. With limited R&D resources, China mobilized all domestic research units at different levels and departments to develop artemisinin collaboratively. The discovery of artemisinin not only

Advances in Parasitology, Volume 116
ISSN 0065-308X
https://doi.org/10.1016/bs.apar.2022.01.002

based on valuable experiential wisdom of traditional medicine, but also relied on excellent synergy among all units. In this study, we reviewed the story of how artemisinin was discovered in China, summarized key factors for new drug development from traditional medicines under limited resources, and raised suggestions to utilize traditional medicines in low- and middle-income countries. This case suggested that the vitality of traditional medicine could be extended by promoting new drug development based on modern methods and collaboration.

Abbreviations

R&D low- and middle-income countries (LMIC) research and development
TCM traditional Chinese medicines
CACMS China Academy of Chinese Medical Sciences
CCAMMS China Academy of Military Medical Sciences
WHO World Health Organization

1. Introduction

Traditional medicines were developed on the basis of indigenous experiences from different cultures within a local environment (Abbo et al., 2019). The ancient and culture-bound traditional medicine practice has benefited human health for thousands of years (Zhu et al., 2016). In 2001, World Health Organization (WHO) released a world review on traditional medicine and acknowledged the contribution of traditional medicine to health care in low- and middle-income countries (LMIC) (Programme On Traditional Medicine, 2001). In 2019, Traditional Chinese Medicine (TCM) was integrated into the ICD-11 system, demonstrating that WHO was stimulating further research, and recognition of TCM worldwide (Lam et al., 2019). Evidence showed that increasing demand was found in Africa, Europe, Asia and America, but the research and development (R&D) of traditional medicine was in early stage around the world (Abdullahi, 2011). Traditional medicines were widely used in China based on medical evidences from increasing scientific studies (Li et al., 2020). With the help of globalization, several TCMs have been modernized and contributed to a wide population range, which accumulated valuable experiences for developing other traditional medicines.

Artemisinin was discovered in 1970s by a Chinese scientist, Prof. Youyou Tu and her team, and known for malaria therapy that has saved millions across the globe. Based on this gift from TCM, many artemisinin-based derivatives were furthered industrialized and adopted to treat malaria patients (Tu, 2011). Artemisinin-based combination therapy was acknowledged by WHO in the Guidelines for the treatment of malaria since 2006 and have save millions of lives worldwide (World Health Organization, 2006). Taking the discovery of artemisinin as an example, this study aimed to summarize the key factors in R&D of traditional medicine under low-resource settings and promote the vitality of traditional medicine in LMIC.

2. Global and Chinese background

2.1 Global malaria burden in 1960s

More than 90% of the global malaria burden centred on African Region nowadays, but in 1960s, Asia and South America were also greatly suffered from malaria (World Health Organization, 2020). In 1965, the malaria endemic area covered 36.65% of the total global land area. The number of people exposed to malaria was around 2 billion, accounting for 57.21% of the global population (Hay et al., 2004). With the widespread use of quinine, quinoline, chloroquine and other conventional antimalarial drugs, resistance became more serious in the 1950s (Wang et al., 2019). Therefore, the Global Malaria Eradication Programme was hindered and ended in 1969. In the following decades, malaria resurged in many parts of the world, especially in Africa (World Health Organization, 2020). Developing a new drug became imperative to save lives threatened by resistant type of malaria.

2.2 Urgent need during wartime

In 1964, the Vietnam War broke out. The non-combat attrition of Vietnamese troops owing to malaria far exceeded the casualties owing to fighting (Liu, 2017). As for the U.S. military, 1% of U.S. combat troops were suffered from malaria each day. According to data published after the Vietnam War, within the 9 years from 1964 to 1973, there were 24,606 U.S. soldiers infected with malaria in Vietnam and an estimated 391,965 sick-days resulting from malaria (Beadle and Hoffman, 1993). Finding alternative drugs for malaria became the decisive factor of this battle. The Republic of Korea sent more than 300,000 soldiers and tens of thousands of civilians to Vietnam to support opposition to the Vietnam War led by the United States. Kim Doo Hie, a preventive medicine specialist affiliated with the National Medical Comprehensive Laboratory, identified the incidence rate of malaria in various units throughout

Vietnam. The results showed that although the Korean army was instructed to take a single weekly dose of chloroquine as a preventive drug and to use repellent and mosquito nets, the incidence rate of malaria remained very high at 11.1%. The only reasonable inference was that the drugs were losing their effectiveness. As a result, South Korean forces began to use chloroquine in combination with other drugs, including dapsone (Harrison and Yim, 2017).

In response to growing drug resistance of malaria, the Walter Reed Army Institute of Research launched a program to find alternative drugs under the political instruction from the U.S. government. Due to the size and urgency of the task, 175 external contractors were involved in its collaborative research. More than 250,000 potential antimalaria compounds were screened and two of them were finally marketed (mefloquine and halofantrine) (Croft, 2007).

In response to growing drug resistance of malaria, the Walter Reed Army Institute of Research in the US launched a program to find alternative drugs, which were the precursors of mefloquine. At the same time, the Vietnamese sought help from China and received fully support from Chairman Mao Zedong. The researches on antimalarial drugs started on May 23, 1967, which was named as "Project 523".

2.3 China's low-resource status

As one of LMIC, the social and economic development of China in 1960s were far more behind developed countries. The China's GDP per capita was $1050 during the 1960s, which was lower than that of East Asia ($1607) and far lower than the average global figure ($4868) (Roser, 2013). The life expectancy at birth in 1960 was only 43.7 years (Roser et al., 2013). In 1970, the health care service facilities were relatively scarce in China. For example, the number of medical doctors per 1000 people was only 0.86 in China, while there was 1.1 in Japan at the same period; the number of hospital beds per 1000 people was 1.54, while there was 12.5 in Japan at the same period. As for the status of population health, in 1960, life expectancy at birth of Chinese people was 43.35 years (National Health Commission of the People's Republic Of China, 1990). During the 1960s, several epidemic, infectious, endemic, and occupational diseases had been effectively controlled (e.g. plague was largely eradicated).

China was lack of health resources and well-established drug supervision system in the 1960s. The health system in China could be divided into four subsystems (Cui, 2021): Three levels of health service institutions, including municipal and district hospitals, community outpatient departments, and health epidemic surveillance system; Prevention-oriented public health system, including institutions dedicated to health and epidemic prevention, endemic disease prevention and control, border health and quarantine, as well as the Patriotic Health Movement Committee; Medical security system covering urban and rural areas, including labour insurance system, socialized medicine, and cooperative medical services; Drug system, including Traditional Chinese Medicine and Western Medicine. The national pharmaceutical industry was under the leadership of a state-owned enterprise named the Chinese Pharmaceutical Company. The drug administration system and patent system had not yet been established in China in 1960s. There were four main health objectives set up by China: Emphasizing prevention; Treating workers, peasants, and soldiers; Integrating Traditional Chinese Medicine and Western medicine; Making health an individual and collective responsibility.

The diplomatic situation made it difficult for China to access international resources and global standards for drug R&D. In 1949, the People's Republic of China established diplomatic relations with the Soviet Union and countries in Eastern Europe such as Bulgaria, Hungary, the Czech Republic, and Poland. From 1960s to 1970s, China's relations with Western countries also developed to a certain extent, and some breakthroughs were made in international health cooperation. In 1963, the Chinese government was invited to send a first medical team to Algeria, which was the starting point of China's health diplomacy. In 1971 and 1972, the People's Republic of China won back its legitimate seats at the UN and the WHO in succession (International Cooperation Division Of National Health Commission, 2019).

3. Research and development history of artemisinin

During the 1960s, the US was involved in the Vietnam War and sent troops to Vietnam beginning in 1961. Malaria was a serious infectious disease in Vietnam and caused massive depletion of military combatants on both sides. At that time, the mortality rate of *P. falciparum* malaria, mainly featuring cerebral malaria, was very high and current antimalarial drugs at the time such as chloroquine, pyrimethamine, proguanil, and quinacrine had poor effectiveness. Therefore, effective antimalaria drugs became an important factor influencing the outcome of the war. Evidence showed that in 1965, the annual incidence rate of malaria among US military personnel stationed in Vietnam was 48.5 per 1000 soldiers per year (Porter, 2006). The US military established a malaria committee to increase funding for malaria research and organized dozens of research institutions to participate in malaria research.

The troops from Democratic Republic of Vietnam has also been severely affected by malaria when they fought in southern areas, so they sought for help from the People's Republic of China for lacking effective measure to solve malaria, which was agreed by Chinese leaders. The researches on antimalarial drugs started on May 23, 1967, which was named as "Project 523". Artemisinin researches were implemented under the leadership of the "Project 523" office. Dozens of research institutions were organized by National 523 Office and Provincial 523 offices, including scientific research centers, medical colleges, and pharmaceutical manufacturing facilities in several provinces. The research span was from the establishment of "Project 523" in 1967 to the artemisinin appraisal conference in 1978 (Li and Zhang, 2020). Based on the accumulated experience from TCM and productive synergy among multiple departments, China discovered the amazing effectiveness of artemisinin as a novel cure against malaria. The key factors in R&D of artemisinin were summarized as four main aspects.

3.1 Establishing a cross-department and cross-region collaboration system

To keep soldiers of the Democratic Republic of Vietnam from malaria, China made massive efforts to search for new drugs. An emergency prevention program was initially managed by the Chinese Academy of Military Medical Sciences to provide instant help for Vietnam. Later, a systematic collaboration among six departments came into being, with the aim to develop effective antimalarial tools.

3.1.1 Emergency prevention program

To meet the urgent needs of malaria prevention, in 1966, the Chinese Academy of Military Medical Sciences developed Antimalarial Tablet No. 1 (pyrimethamine + dapsone) as an emergency preventive prescription drug. To extend the protective period to 10–14 days, Antimalarial Tablet No. 2 (pyrimethamine + weekly sulfanilamide) was developed in 1967. In 1969, the Second Military Medical University and Shanghai Institute of Pharmaceutical Industry jointly developed Antimalarial Tablet No. 3 containing piperaquine phosphate, to be taken once monthly (Zhang, 2018).

3.1.2 Systematic collaboration of multi-sectors (departments, provinces and research groups)

In 1966, China Academy of Military Medical Sciences (CCAMMS) drafted the *Three-Year Research Plan (Protocol)* after field investigations in Vietnam, with reference to the domestic and international literature. With approval of the State Council, the State Scientific and Technological Commission and General Logistics Department of Chinese People's Liberation Army held a national collaborative conference in Beijing entitled "Research on antimalaria drugs" on May 23, 1967. Leaders from relevant ministries, military headquarters, and from different provinces, cities, and military regions participated in this conference. As an emergency military project for foreign aid, the Project 523 was officially launched.

To implement Project 523, the national leadership group for malaria control and prevention drug research (referred to as National 523 Office) was established after the collaborative conference to take charge of research plan implementation and collaboration among regions and departments. The National 523 Office was composed of six sectors, including the State Scientific and Technological Commission, the General Logistics Department of Chinese People's Liberation Army, Science, Technology and Industry Commission for National Defense, Ministry of Health, Ministry of Chemical Industry, and the Chinese Academy of Sciences (Fig. 1). Each sector would designate focal points to be responsible for communication with National 523 Offices and implementation of all tasks in their subordinate units in a timely manner.

Subordinate units of the six departments established regional 523 research groups and offices in Beijing, Shanghai, Guangdong, Yunnan,

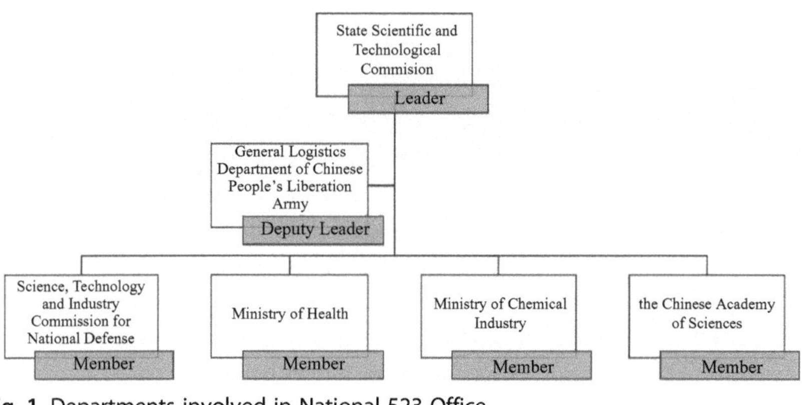

Fig. 1 Departments involved in National 523 Office.

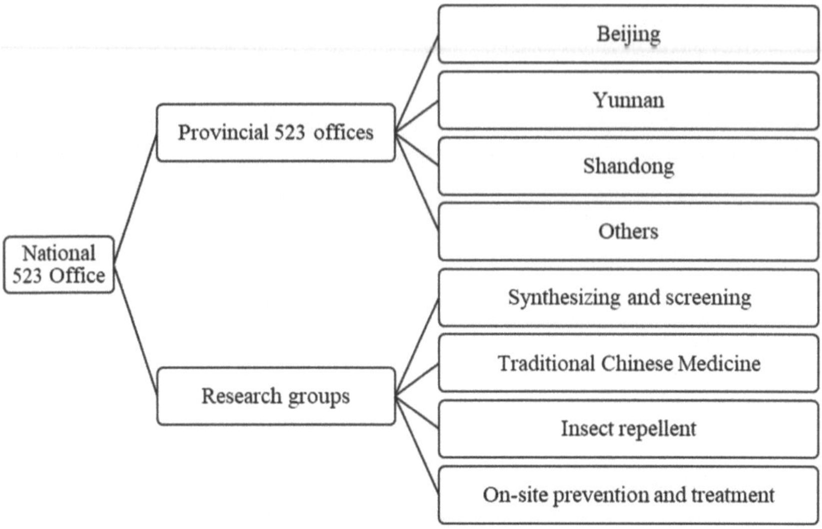

Fig. 2 Task assignment of National 523 Office.

Sichuan, Guangxi, and other provinces. These offices were responsible for supervising the implementation of the regional research plan and daily contact between upper and lower levels.

Four research groups were established according to different research directions, including chemical synthesizing and screening, Traditional Chinese Medicine, insect repellent development, and on-site prevention and treatment (Fig. 2). Later, successive groups were established focused on acupuncture, treatment of *P. falciparum* malaria, malaria immunity, and mosquito-repelling agents and equipment. Each group was responsible for implementing professional research plans and conducting academic and technical information exchanges (Zhang, 2018).

3.2 Exploring traditional medicine by modern methods

With profound knowledge of traditional medicine, China had an advantage in developing novel antimalarial drugs. Based on TCM books and folk recipes, Chinese scientists screened over 40,000 herbs and compounds. The TCM research group led by Youyou Tu organized more than 640 recipes. The scientific research teams in Beijing, Guangdong, Guangxi, Sichuan, Yunnan, Jiangsu and other regions also performed in-depth investigations to collect folk remedies. Modern drug development process was adopted in these researches, including extracting active components, safety testing in the laboratory and clinical research (Fig. 3) (U.S. Food and Administration, 2018).

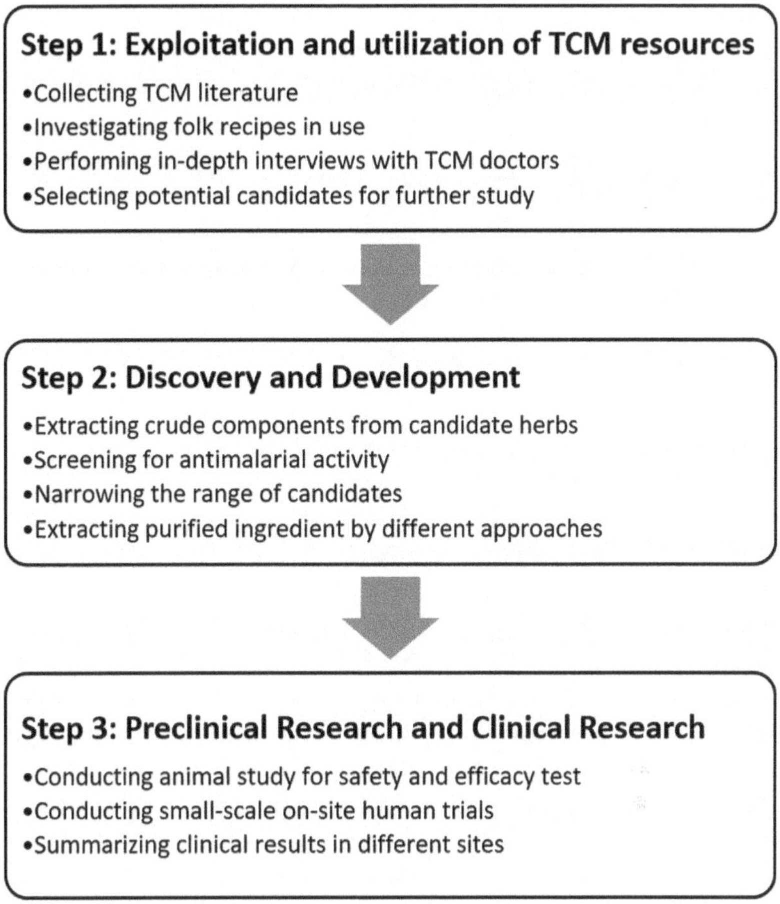

Fig. 3 Exploration flow of antimalarial drugs on the basis of TCM.

After concluding the current evidence, 10 key herbs including Changshan (Chinese name of antifebrile dichroa root), Yingzhao (Chinese name of *Ar. hexapetalus*) and Qinghao (Chinese name of *Artemisia annua* Linn) were selected for further research (Su and Miller, 2015).

3.2.1 Research on Changshan

At the early stage of TCM investigation, Changshan was considered as an important candidate because of its good antimalarial effects. In Beijing, China Academy of Chinese Medical Sciences (CACMS), CCAMMS and Beijing Pharmaceutical Factory jointly conducted researches and successfully synthesized febrifugine, the active ingredients of Changshan. Later, they modified its chemical structure to lighten side effects of vomiting and developed a series of derivatives, among which a compound with high potency (named 7002) was selected. After a pharmacological toxicity study, a clinical trial was carried out in Hainan from 1970 to 1973. However, toxic side effects persisted and the incidence of vomiting remained high. Therefore, studies on Changshan were finally terminated in Beijing.

Sichuan Institute of TCM undertook a number of research tasks involving Changshan and febrifugine. Sichuan Medical College, Chengdu University of TCM and other organizations conducted further researches on reducing side effects, but the results were not promising. Even so, the researches on Changshan provided a good example for Qinghao (Zhang, 2015).

3.2.2 Research on Yingzhao

From 1967 to 1969, National and Provincial 523 offices established investigation teams to find potential antimalarial herbs in Yunnan, Guangdong, Jiangsu, and other regions. After preliminary study, another herb named Yingzhao was discovered as a candidate. In 1969, CACMS, Zhongshan School of Medicine, Sun Yat-Sen University carried out a study on the antimalarial effect of Yingzhao. Its active ingredient was named Yingzhaosu A, which had strong antimalarial effects. However, the resources of Yingzhao was scarce and the content of effective components was quite low. Therefore, it was difficult to extract active ingredients in large quantities. Through cooperation with the Department of Chemistry, Sun Yat-Sen University, it was determined that the chemical structure of Yingzhaosu was a fat-soluble sesquiterpene with bears a peroxide grouping, which greatly inspired the work on determining the chemical structure of artemisinin (Zhang, 2018).

3.2.3 Breakthrough in antimalarial effect of Qinghao

Qinghao has been used for more than 2000 years in China. Qinghao has the effects of clearing deficient heat, eliminating hectic fever, relieving summer heat, preventing malaria, and abating jaundice. The first use of Qinghao was to treat haemorrhoids, according to the silk manuscript *Prescription for 52 Diseases,* unearthed from tomb No. 3 of Mawangdui (168 BC, the 12th year of Emperor Wendi of the Han Dynasty). During the Eastern Jin Dynasty (about 400 AC), the antimalarial effects of Qinghao was recorded in Ge Hong's "A Handbook of Prescriptions for Emergencies". The recipe was "A handful of Qinghao immersed in 2 L of water, wring out the juice, and drink it all" (Tan et al., 2020).

In the investigation of folk remedies, the researchers in Nanjing learned that in 1969, rural doctors and residents of Gaoyou County in Jiangsu Province used local Qinghao to treat and prevent malaria, which achieved good results. A folk song said that "Don't worry after contracting malaria. Take brown sugar and Qinghao". In early 1970s, CAMMS and CACMS decided to send Guoming Gu and Yagang Yu to screening effective herbs for mouse malaria. Based on the *Malaria Album* published by Shanghai Science and Technology Press in 1965, as well as records of "Malaria Phylum" in the *Complete Records of Ancient and Modern Medical Works of the Grand Compendium of Books*, they selected Chinese medicines with records of malaria prevention that appeared frequently in single prescription and compound prescription forms.

In June 1970, the report "Literature on formulas and medicines for malaria treatment" was published. This publication described eight key Chinese herbs including Qinghao which were worthy of further investigation in animal studies, because all these herbs appeared in records of single prescription and also frequently applied in compound prescriptions. After water decoction and alcohol extraction in the laboratory, the extraction from each herb were sent to Xiuqing Jiao's team at the Institute of Microbiology and Epidemiology, Academy of Military Medical Sciences, for conducting trials against mouse malaria. Among these, the ethanol extraction of Qinghao had a good antimalarial effect, with an inhibition rate of 60–80% against mouse malaria in several experiments. According to the results of field investigations in Gaoyou and Yagang Yu's work, Youyou Tu and other researchers re-screened Qinghao, which had a high inhibition rate of mouse malaria. They followed basic techniques in selecting solvents, such as water, alcohol and ethyl ether, during the extraction of effective components of Chinese herbal medicines. Inspired by Ge Hong's "A Handbook of Prescriptions for Emergencies", she assumed that extraction methods of boiling might damage the active ingredient and used low-temperature ethyl ether extraction at lower temperature. After removing an acidic portion, the low-temperature ethyl ether extract of Qinghao showed 100% inhibition in the test against mouse malaria, *Plasmodium berghei* (Miller and Su, 2011).

3.3 Promoting synergy through efficient information-sharing mechanisms

The research abilities of Chinese research centers were insufficient to complete drug R&D on their own. In the early 1970s, research centers in three provinces had different breakthroughs. Under coordination of National 523 office, different research centers shared their latest progress in a timely manner through regular meetings and visits, which greatly promoted artemisinin R&D (Zhang et al., 2017).

3.3.1 Information-sharing and arrangement at national level

The State Council and Central Military Commission of Chinese Communist Party issued a notice calling for strengthening of the leadership of Project 523. Thus, the Ministry of Health became the leader of National 523 office in May 1971. In March 1972, the National 523 Office held a meeting of two professional groups (hereinafter referred to as Nanjing Conference) on chemical synthetic drugs and TCM in Nanjing. At a meeting of TCM research group, Youyou Tu, on behalf of Beijing Institute of TCM (a subordinate institute of CACMS), reported the recent results regarding the inhibition rate of Qinghao extraction against mouse malaria of nearly 100%. The 523 office and professional group thus attached great importance to the effect of low-temperature ethyl ether extraction of Qinghao (Huang and Zhu, 2012).

3.3.2 Extracting active ingredients in Beijing

In 1972, National 523 office assigned Beijing Institute of TCM to carry out research on separating out the purified effective antimalarial ingredient of Qinghao. Different approaches were adopted, for example, alumina column chromatography was used but no valuable ingredients could be obtained. To separate neutral compounds, a method of gradient elution in which petroleum ether and ethyl acetate petroleum ether solution was poured onto silica gel column was adopted in November 1972. In this way, three ingredients were separated out, named crystal I, crystal II, and crystal III. By conducting trials against mouse malaria, Zuguang Ye proved that crystal II had antimalarial effects (renamed Artemisinin II later). So as to get Artemisinin II into clinical trials as soon as possible, shortly after toxicity testing in mice, three researchers took Artemisinin II voluntarily, and found no obvious change in physiological indexes such as heart, brain, liver, kidney, or blood. Thus, leaders of Beijing Institute of TCM agreed to carry out clinical trials of Artemisinin II.

From September to October in 1973, a clinical trial of Artemisinin II was carried out in Changjiang County, Hainan Province, which turned out to be unsatisfactory. In the clinical trial, a clinical symptom of premature ventricular beats appeared in two patients with *P. falciparum* malaria. From 1973 to 1974, research on Artemisinin II at Beijing Institute of TCM remained stagnant (Zhang, 2018), but its timely information-sharing on active ingredients and the spirit of dedication to science inspired the research in other organizations.

3.3.3 Promising antimalarial effects of Huanghuahao extract in Shandong

After Nanjing Conference, representatives of Shandong Institute of Parasitic Diseases underwent training at Beijing Institute of TCM. Based on the experience of Beijing Institute of TCM, Zhenxing Wei's team used Huanghuahao extract (Huanghuahao was another species of Qinghao in local areas and was collectively referred to as "artemisinin" after 1978) in toxicity testing against mouse malaria and found consistent result with Beijing Institute of TCM. On October 21, 1972, they reported to National 523 office that the results were consistent with Beijing Institute of TCM. In 1973, the Shandong Institute of Parasitic Diseases and Shandong Institute of Chinese Medicine carried out clinical trials of low-temperature ethyl ether extract from Huanghuahao among 30 patients with *P. vivax* malaria in Juye County. The results of the clinical trials proved that treatment with six capsules (each capsule equivalent to 17.1 g crude extract from Huanghuahao) over 3 days showed a strong killing effect on *P. vivax*, with no obvious side effects (Zhang et al., 2017). To understand the specific research progress in Shandong and exchange research experiences, the National 523 Office arranged an visit to Shandong and discussed the latest advances, especially in regard of cardiotoxicity and temperature control in extraction process.

3.3.4 Improving raw material resources and extraction method in Yunnan

At the end of 1972, Liangshu Fu, director of Kunming 523 Office, travelled to Beijing to attend meetings and learned about the research progress regarding Qinghao. He returned to Kunming and conveyed the news to 523 research groups in Yunnan Institute of Materia Medica. At the beginning of 1973, Luo Zeyuan from Yunnan Institute of Materia Medica collected some *An. ordosica* (later identified as the macrocephalic variant of *An. annua* L.)

from Yunnan University, which was extracted with petroleum ether, ethyl ether, ethyl acetate, and methanol. Later, researchers carried out malaria inhibition testing in mice using these extracts. In April 1973, ethyl ether extract was found to be effective against mouse malaria and tentatively named "Ku Hao crystal III" (later called "Huanghaosu"). By October 1973, Yunnan Institute of Materia Medica had completed the malaria inhibition tests in mice and pharmacological toxicity testing of Huanghaosu, and no obvious harm to animals was observed (Zhang, 2018).

It is worth mentioning that in 1973, Yunnan Institute of Materia Medica found that there were few local sources of *A. annua* L., which yielded very low extraction and crystallization efficiency. In the summer of 1973, a batch of *A. annua* L. was purchased from the Youyang area of Chongqing City, with a content of *A. annua* L. 10 times that of *A. macrocephala*. In 1974, researchers of Yunnan Institute of Materia Medica adopted solvent gasoline for cold soaking and concentration to obtain Huanghaosu. Then it was then recrystallized with 50% ethanol to obtain the pure product. This extraction method was called the "solvent gasoline method" and provided sufficient Huanghaosu for subsequent experiments in Yunnan Province, which greatly accelerated research progress. In the autumn of 1973, Zhou Keding, head of National 523 Office, and researchers from Beijing Institute of TCM went to Yunnan Institute of Materia Medica to learn about the research progress on Qinghao and the advanced extraction methods used in Yunnan Province, which were brought back as reference material. The solvent gasoline method was still used to extract artemisinin in industrial-scale production nowadays (Li and Zhang, 2020). Meanwhile, this provided a basis for identifying Youyang as an area with high-quality *A. annua* L. Since 1975, all institutes in Project 523 began to buy *A. annua* L. from Youyang as the main source of Qinghao.

3.4 National cooperation in overcoming challenge of artemisinin production

The industrial production of artemisinin required technological support from other departments. To overcome the challenge of producing artemisinin, the National 523 Office arranged for additional cooperation among institutions, medical colleges, and private enterprises (Tu et al., 2015).

3.4.1 Task arrangement by National 523 office

On February 28, 1974, a symposium on artemisinin research was held at Beijing Institute of TC. Research institutions in Beijing, Shandong, and

Yunnan all sent relevant researchers to participate. After exchange of research results on Qinghao at different institutions, the division of tasks was discussed. The main contents were as follows: (1) It was suggested that Beijing Institute of TCM should cooperate with relevant institutions in Shanghai to clarify the chemical structure of Qinghao extraction; (2) Improvement of the extraction technology for effective ingredient of Qinghao and investigation on collection, harvest, resources of Qinghao should be carried out with reference to local conditions in three provinces; (3) Clinical observation among 150–200 individuals to assess effective ingredient of Qinghao should be completed by October 1974; this was mainly the responsibility of Shandong Institute of Parasitic Diseases and Institute of Malignant Malaria Prevention. Other institutions should send relevant researchers to participate.

In February 1975, the National 523 Office held a meeting at Beijing Beiwei Road Hotel (hereinafter referred to as the Beijing Conference), to which responsible persons of all 523 offices and some institutions undertaking related tasks were invited. A researcher from Guangdong 523 research group reported "A summary of 18 cases of malaria treated with artemisinin". This report was based on the clinical trials in Yunnan and concluded by Guoqiao Li's team. At the meeting, it was concluded that experimental research on Qinghao and its extracts during the past 3 years had been very promising and should be undertaken as a key project to carry out by comprehensive and in-depth research. This was listed as the focus of 523 tasks in 1975. In April 1975, according to arrangements made at the Beijing Conference, the National 523 Office held another national conference on Chinese herbal medicine research in Chengdu, Sichuan Province (hereinafter referred to as the Chengdu Conference). Scientific and technological researchers and leaders from 39 units affiliated with relevant ministries, commissions, military headquarters, and military regions attended the meeting. Research progress on Qinghao and artemisinin was reported by the various research institutions. The following research direction was proposed at the meeting: (1) Research on simple preparations of Qinghao should be carried out as soon as possible. (2) Research of artemisinin should focus on improving its curative effect, reducing the reignition rate, and improving the production process. (3) Comprehensive and systematic research should be carried out on resource investigation, extraction methods, pharmacology and toxicology, improvement of dosage forms, quality standards, in-vivo metabolism, and chemical structure determination and transformation (Zhang, 2018).

3.4.2 Clinical research conducted by medical colleges

From May to October 1974, Shandong Institute of Chinese Medicine, Institute of Parasitic Diseases, and Qingdao Medical College formed a cooperative group on Qinghao. A total of 26 patients with *P. vivax* malaria in Juye County were treated and observed. The total amount of drug used was 0.6–1.2g, and treatment lasted for 3 days. The conclusion was that artemisinin was a good, quick-acting antimalarial drug, and no obvious side effects were observed. However, there was a high rate of short-term relapse after drug withdrawal. From September to October 1974, the clinical cooperation group of Yunnan Province took artemisinin provided by Yunnan Institute of Materia Medica to Fengqing County and Yun County in Yunnan Province to observe the clinical effect on *P. falciparum* malaria. Owing to the small number of patients admitted locally, the progress was not smooth. At that time, Jianfang Zhang, deputy director of National 523 Office, went to Yunnan to follow up on the work and learned that *P. falciparum* malaria was prevalent in the Gengma area and there were many patients with cerebral malaria. He suggested that Guoqiao Li's group from Guangzhou College of Chinese Medicine, which was carrying out research on the treatment of cerebral malaria locally, undertook the task of artemisinin clinical trials in Gengma area. In November, the staff of Yunnan Institute of Materia Medica and the Institute for Malaria Control, as well as observers from the Beijing Institute of TCM, took artemisinin to the People's Hospital of Gengma County and delivered it to Guoqiao Li's team for clinical trials. After treating 18 patients with malaria (including 14 with *P. falciparum* malaria), the results showed that the killing effect of artemisinin on *P. falciparum* was faster than that of chloroquine. However, there were also some problems, such as reproduction of *Plasmodium* and recurrence of symptoms. Nevertheless, efficacy and safety of artemisinin in the treatment of *P. falciparum* malaria in tropical areas was basically evaluated as positive.

It was worth mentioning that Guoqiao Li successfully treated three patients with cerebral malaria, including one pregnant woman. This clinical treatment provided convincing observation data, leading to the conclusion that treatment of dangerous *P. falciparum* malaria with artemisinin had a quick effect, high short-term efficacy, low toxicity, but high recurrence rate.

3.4.3 Structural determination conducted by research institutions

The structural analysis and identification of artemisinin began in 1972, after animal antimalaria experiments using crude extract of Qinghao were carried out by Beijing Institute of TCM. Beijing Institute of TCM invited external units to carry out elemental analysis, low resolution mass spectrometry, and nuclear magnetic resonance spectroscopy. Professor Qishou Lin of Beijing Medical College speculated that artemisinin might belong to the sesquiterpenoids. Later, in 1973, Beijing Institute of TCM proposed cooperation with Shanghai Institute of Organic Chemistry which had experience with terpenoids, to determine the chemical structure as soon as possible. In 1974, Beijing Institute of TCM sent a researcher to Shanghai Institute of Organic Chemistry to cooperate in researching the chemical structure of artemisinin. In 1974, Keding Zhou, director of the 523 office, invited experts in structural biology from the Institute of Biophysics, Chinese Academy of Sciences to participate in the collaboration, hoping to use its four-circle X-ray diffractometer. In 1975, Shanghai Institute of Organic Chemistry proposed that the possible structural formula of artemisinin contained lactone peroxide, referring to the peroxide grouping in Yingzhaosu A and the structure of Artemisinin II isolated from Qinghao. Later, the researchers used the four-circle X-ray diffractometer to collect accurate diffraction intensity data. They confirmed that the chemical structure of artemisinin was a new sesquiterpene lactone that had never been seen before. After that, Institute of Biophysics determined the absolute configuration of artemisinin (Liang, 2017).

3.4.4 Research on resources and preparation

In 1972, Gaoyou County established an Qinghao malaria control verification group, which was composed of the Health Bureau, epidemic prevention station, and Cheluo District Hospital. Qinghao's antimalarial effects were explored in trials, including fresh Qinghao juice, boiling agents, decoction, pills, tablets, and other dosage forms. The verification group summarized the six kinds of preparations used in recent years and selected an extract tablet with the advantages of being a rapid antipyretic with a rapid malaria negative conversion time, high cure rate, and low recurrence rate. From June to October 1976, Qinghao was administered to more than 240,000 people at 26 observation points in the five experimental areas of Gaoyou County to prevent malaria, with incidence dropping by 50% compared with the same period in 1975. Another 201 cases were treated with Qinghao and the effective rate was 89%. During this period, Beijing Institute of TCM sent two researchers to Gaoyou to help carry out the research and application of a simple preparation of Qinghao.

From February 18 to 28, 1977, researchers from 15 units including pharmaceutical institute, botanical institute, drug control institute, parasitic disease institute, and pharmaceutical manufacturing facilities attended the first exchange course on Qinghao content determination. A variety of content determination methods established by the researchers were discussed. Ultraviolet spectrophotometry was considered the superior method. In September 1977, the second seminar on content determination was held, where it was finally agreed that ultraviolet spectrophotometry was the best method. Based on these findings, the content determination method and quality standards of Qinghao were drafted.

3.5 Disclosure of artemisinin by Chinese government and scientists

Domestic trial application of artemisinin began in 1973. Several institutes and departments launched clinical trials to evaluate the safety and efficacy of artemisinin. In 1978, the artemisinin appraisal conference was held by National 523 office to declare the scientific achievement of discovering a new antimalarial drug, artemisinin. Chinese scientists first disclosed the chemical structure of artemisinin. According to the record of this conference, until November in 1978, Chinese institutes had carried out clinical research on artemisinin among thousands of malaria cases, and the results for both *P. falciparum* and *P. vivax* were promising.

International application of artemisinin began in Cambodia rather than Vietnam. In 1975, China sent an investigative group to Cambodia, for malaria prevention and control. Artemisinin was brought to Cambodia in the form of oil-and-water suspension injections prepared by Shandong Institute of Traditional Chinese Medicine and Yunnan Institute of Medicine. In half a year, more than 4700 patients with malaria and 43 critically ill patients were successfully treated with artemisinin.

3.5.1 Publication of chemical structure

Chinese scientists were the first to disclose the chemical structure of artemisinin. In 1976, it was learned that a plant chemist in Yugoslavia was also isolating and extracting natural compounds from local *A. annua* L. The researchers in China found that that one compound was the same as artemisinin. Therefore, they decided to publish their research findings in academic journals and to disclose the chemical structure of artemisinin to clarify that artemisinin was discovered by Chinese scientists and win acclaim for their efforts and for the country. The national patent system in China was established after 1985. Therefore, the first paper on artemisinin was published in 1977 in the 3rd issue of *Scientific Bulletin*, entitled "Artemisinin: A New Type of Sesquiterpene Lactone" (The Cooperation Group On Research Of Artemisinin's Structure, 1977). The structural formula of artemisinin was reported, without mentioning the antimalarial efficacy of artemisinin. In 1979, other papers published the structure and configuration of artemisinin consecutively in *Acta Chemica Sinica* and *Science China* (Liu et al., 1979; The Cooperation Group On Research Of Artemisinin's Structure, 1979).

3.5.2 Publication of antimalarial efficacy

In 1979, "Research on the antimalarial drug artemisinin" was published in the *Pharmaceutical Bulletin* (renamed the *Journal of Chinese Medicine*) (The Cooperation Group On Research Of Artemisinin, 1979). This review mainly reported artemisinin's efficacy, toxicology, pharmacodynamics, and clinical trials (artemisinin tablets, oil solution, oil suspension agents, and water suspension agents). The English version of this article was published in 1979 in the 12th issue of the *Chinese Medical Journal* (p. 811–816). In 1980, the report "Research on artemisinin derivatives" was published in the fourth issue of the *Pharmaceutical Sciences Bulletin,* which reported the clinical effects of SM 804 (sodium artesunate) in 186 cases. Later, several English Journal also published the discovery of artemisinin (Hien and White, 1993; Klayman, 1985). These publications drew worldwide attention and interest in this new drug, which resulted in international collaboration on the development of artemisinin antimalarials.

4. Conclusions and perspectives

4.1 Conclusions

Traditional medicines are generated from the medical practice of human being in different parts of the world and reflected human wisdom in the past thousands of years. China's discovery of artemisinin set an example to explore traditional medicine under low-resource settings. In this study, we reviewed the story of how artemisinin was discovered in China. Due to the limited R&D resources in the 1970s, China adopted a collaborative way to develop artemisinin involving all domestic research units at different levels and departments. The inspiration from traditional medicine and excellent synergy among all units led to China's outstanding contribution to innovative antimalarial drugs, namely artemisinin. The discovery of artemisinin highlighted that LMICs should strengthen the utilization of traditional medicine, integrate traditional medicines with modern drug development standard, establish a systematic R&D model and attach importance to interdisciplinary cooperation.

4.2 Perspectives

There is no doubt that developing traditional medicines could not only promote primary health care, especially in LMIC, but also benefit more people globally through R&D and industrialization. Therefore, following recommendations are put forward:

(1) *Strengthening the utilization of traditional medicine*

The LMICs need to strengthen the utilization of traditional medicine to accelerate new drug development Apart from health perspective, developing new drugs based on traditional medicine can stimulate the growth of pharmaceutical industry and promote regional economic development (Zhu et al., 2017). Many LMICs possessed abundant traditional medicine resources, but the R&D of traditional medicine in most countries were in early stage due to social and economic restrictions (Abdullahi, 2011). The experience from artemisinin's discovery history and the evidence from other studies jointly suggested that the research infrastructure in LMICs should be improved to act as the drug development pipeline (Patwardhan and Mashelkar, 2009).

(2) *Integrating traditional medicines with modern drug development standard*

Under the surveillance of national drug regulatory agency and WHO, all new drug development should be science-based and stick to strict procedures including preclinical studies and three phases of investigational clinical trials (Williams, 2016). Since the regulatory agencies of LMIC had not established thorough standards for new drug approval, Regulation and Prequalification Department of WHO provided clear guidance for related departments and companies. Through participation in the WHO prequalification, new drug from LMIC would be assessed in quality, safety and effectiveness and be able to supply to global market if approved.

(3) *Establishing a systematic R&D model to adapt to low-resource settings*

Several new drugs developed from TCM have been modernized and contributed to a wide population range, including Artemisinin and Yunnan Baiyao. The productive synergy among multiple departments in China promoted the amazing discovery of artemisinin as a novel cure against malaria. Yunnan Baiyao was a famous drug used for trauma treatment and its manufacturer became one of the top 50 Chinese pharmaceutical enterprises (Zhu et al., 2017). These successful cases suggested that under low-resource settings, a government-led R&D pattern including both public and private sectors would be an optimal solution.

(4) *Attaching importance to interdisciplinary cooperation*

New drug development required interdisciplinary knowledge and technology, which were weak in LMIC. Interdisciplinary cooperation and cross-department cooperation should be equally valued. During the discovery of Artemisinin, the cooperation among institutions, medical colleges, and private enterprises were arranged, which included researchers from the fields of medicine, biology, chemistry, physics and so on. This collaboration pattern and research division should be encouraged to release potential for LIMC.

It is desirable that some undiscovered records in traditional medicine might fill gaps in modern medicine and give numerus people hope, but to realize drug innovation, all stakeholders should make joint efforts and establish efficient collaboration mechanism. Also, under the technical guidance from WHO prequalification, the new drug R&D based on traditional medicines would be consistent with current new drug development standard and recognized by global market easily. The discovery of artemisinin in China gave a reliable pattern to promote sustainable development of traditional medicines and a good example to realize R&D of traditional medicine under low-resource countries.

Acknowledgements

This work was supported by Bill & Melinda Gates Foundation (No. INV-018913). We would like to thank National Institute of Parasitic Diseases, China CDC, China for supporting this study.

References

Abbo, C., Odokonyero, R., Ovuga, E., 2019. A narrative analysis of the link between modern medicine and traditional medicine in Africa: a case of mental health in Uganda. Brain Res. Bull. 145, 109–116.

Abdullahi, A.A., 2011. Trends and challenges of traditional medicine in Africa. Afr. J. Tradit. Complement. Altern. Med. 8, 115–123.

Beadle, C., Hoffman, S.L., 1993. History of malaria in the United States Naval forces at war: world war I through the Vietnam conflict. Clin. Infect. Dis. 16, 320–329.

Croft, A.M., 2007. A lesson learnt: the rise and fall of lariam and halfan. J. R. Soc. Med. 100, 170–174.

Cui, J., 2021. Great achievements have been made in health care under the leadership of the party [Dang Ling Dao Wei Sheng Jian Kang Shi Ye Qu De Wei Da Cheng Jiu]. China Health (07), 66–69. https://doi.org/10.15973/j.cnki.cn11-3708/d.2021.07.021.

Food, U.S., Administration, D., 2018. The drug development process 2021. Available: Https://Www.Fda.Gov/Patients/Learn-About-Drug-And-Device-Approvals/Drug-Development-Process [Accessed 2018-01-04].

Harrison, M., Yim, S.V., 2017. War on two fronts: the fight against parasites in Korea and Vietnam. Med. Hist. 61, 401–423.

Hay, S.I., Guerra, C.A., Tatem, A.J., Noor, A.M., Snow, R.W., 2004. The global distribution and population at risk of malaria: past, present, and future. Lancet Infect. Dis. 4, 327–336.

Hien, T.T., White, N.J., 1993. Qinghaosu. Lancet 341, 603–608.

Huang, S., Zhu, Y., 2012. Inventor's right of science and technology and resolution of the Debate Over Tu Youyou's invention of artemisinin. In: Studies in Dialectics of Nature. vol. 28, pp. 86–90.

International Cooperation Division of National Health Commission, 2019. Progress and achievements in international health cooperation and exchanges in the past 70 years in P.R. China. Chinese Health Resources 22 (4), 251–253.

Klayman, D.L., 1985. Qinghaosu (Artemisinin): an antimalarial drug from China. Science 228, 1049–1055.

Lam, W.C., Lyu, A., Bian, Z., 2019. Icd-11: impact on traditional Chinese medicine and world healthcare systems. Pharm. Med. 33, 373–377.

Li, R., Zhang, D., 2020. The search for antimalarial drugs and the discovery of artemisinin. Chinese Ann. Hist. Sci. Technol. 2, 073–134.

Li, Q., Wang, H., Li, X., Zheng, Y., Wei, Y., Zhang, P., Ding, Q., Lin, J., Tang, S., Zhao, Y., Zhao, L., Tong, X., 2020. The role played by traditional Chinese medicine in preventing and treating Covid-19 in China. Front. Med. 14, 681–688.

Liang, L., 2017. Historical review of artemisinin molecular and structure determination [Qinghaosu Fen Zi He Li Ti Jie Gou Ce Ding De Li Shi Hui Gu]. Prog. Biochem. Biophys. 44, 6–16.

Liu, B., 2017. Artemisinin: the scientific achievements resulted from the Vietnam war [Qinghaosu: Yue Zhan Cui Sheng De Ke Yan Cheng Guo]. Cult. Hist Vis [Wen Shi Bo Lan] (9), 16–17.

Liu, J., Ni, M., Fan, J., Youyou, T., Zhaohua, W., Yulin, W., Weishan, Z., 1979. The structure and reaction of artemisinin [Qinghaosu De Jie Gou Yu Fan Ying]. Acta Chem. Sin. 37 (02), 129–143.

Miller, L.H., Su, X., 2011. Artemisinin: discovery from the Chinese herbal garden. Cell 146, 855–858.

National Health Commission of the People's Republic Of China, 1990. Health Statistics Yearbook. 1960. National Health Commission of the People's Republic of China, Beijing.

Patwardhan, B., Mashelkar, R.A., 2009. Traditional medicine-inspired approaches to drug discovery: can ayurveda show the way forward? Drug Discov. Today 14, 804–811.

Porter, W.D., 2006. Imported malaria and conflict: 50 years of experience in the U.S. Military. Mil. Med. 171, 925–928.

Programme On Traditional Medicine, 2001. Legal status of traditional medicine and complementary/alternative medicine: a worldwide review. World Health Organization, Geneva.

Roser, M., 2013. *Economic growth* [Online]. Online at Ourworldindata.Org: Our World in Data. Available: Https://Ourworldindata.Org/Economic-Growth. (Accessed).

Roser, M., Ortiz-Ospina, E., Ritchie, H., 2013. Life expectancy. Available:. Https://Ourworldindata.Org/Life-Expectancy [Accessed 2021-06-25].

Su, X.Z., Miller, L.H., 2015. The Discovery Of Artemisinin And The Nobel Prize in physiology or medicine. Sci. China Life Sci. 58, 1175–1179.
Tan, J., Wan, F., Tan, C., 2020. The application history of Qinghao as medicine and food [Qinghao Yao Yong Shi Yong Li Shi Kao Lue]. Asia-Pac. Tradit. Med. 16, 75–76.
The Cooperation Group On Research Of Artemisinin, 1979. Research on a new antimalarial drug: artemisinin. Pharm. Bull. 14, 49–53.
The Cooperation Group On Research Of Artemisinin's Structure, 1977. Artemisinin: a new type of sesquiterpene lactone [Yi Zhong Xin Xing De Bei Ban Tie: Qinghaosu]. Chin. Sci. Bull. 22, 142.
The Cooperation Group On Research Of Artemisinin's Structure, 1979. The crystal structure and absolute configuration of artemisinin. Sci. Sin. 23 (11), 1114–1128.
Tu, Y., 2011. The discovery of artemisinin (Qinghaosu) and gifts from Chinese medicine. Nat. Med. 17, 1217–1220.
Tu, Y., Luo, Z., Li, G., Zhang, J., Wu, Z., Shi, B., Li, R., 2015. Interveiws On 523 project and the discovery of artemisinin [523 Renwu Yu Qinghaosu Yanfa Fangtanlu]. Hunan Education Publishing House, Huan.
Wang, J., Zhu, Y., Xu, C., Yang, J., Qiu, C., Liao, F., Jiang, T., Tu, Y., 2019. Research course and value of artemisinin [Qinghaosu De Yan Jiu Li Cheng Yu Jia Zhi]. Electron. J. Emer. Infect. Dis. 4, 193–195.
Williams, C.T., 2016. Food and drug administration drug approval process: a history and overview. Nurs. Clin. North Am. 51, 1–11.
World Health Organization, 2006. Guidelines for the treatment of malaria. World Health Organization, Geneva.
World Health Organization, 2020. World malaria report 2020. World Health Organization, Geneva.
Zhang, N., 2015. Scientific implications of artemisinin discovery [Qinghaosu Fa Xian De Ke Xue Qi Shi]. Sci. Technol. Rev. 33, 90–92.
Zhang, J., 2018. A late report for project 523: 1967–2017 [Chi Dao De Bao Gao: Zhong Guo 523 Xiang Mu]. Sichuan People's Publishing House, Beijing.
Zhang, D., Li, R., Rao, Y., 2017. Inheritance and innovation: project 523 and artemisinin discovery [Ji Cheng Yu Chuang Xin: 523 Ren Wu Yu Qinghaosu Yan Fa]. China Press for Science and Technology, Beijing.
Zhu, Z., Wang, T., Fu, D., Gui, Y., Wang, J., Cui, T., 2016. Innovative development path of ethnomedicines: an overview of ethnomedicines in China. Front. Med. 10, 166–177.
Zhu, Z., Gui, Y., Wang, L., Wang, T., Yang, Y., Niu, Y., Fu, D., Wang, J., Cui, T., 2017. Innovative development path of ethnomedicines: a case study. Front. Med. 11, 297–305.

FSC
www.fsc.org
MIX
Papier | Fördert
gute Waldnutzung
FSC® C083411

Kolibri 360 GmbH
Ferdinand-Jühlke-Straße 7
99095 Erfurt, Deutschland
produktsicherheit@kolibri360.de